Buyer
—*Be* Wise!

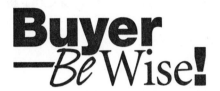

Buyer—Be Wise!

The Consumer's Guide to Buying Quality Nutritional Supplements

by Karolyn A. Gazella

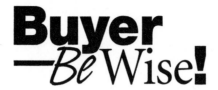

Published by:
IMPAKT Communications, Inc.
P.O. Box 12496
Green Bay, WI 54307-2496
E-mail: impakt@dct.com
Fax: (920) 434-8884
www.impakt.com

Dedication

This book is dedicated to the loving memory of my mom, Eunice Gazella. Everything positive in my life continues to be influenced by her spirit and love.

Acknowledgements

A project like this requires a commitment from several individuals working together for a common cause. I am simply the mouthpiece who delivers the message, and I do not work alone.

The healthcare professionals featured in this book were carefully selected. I am proud to be associated with these experts: Marla Ahlgrimm, R.Ph.; Lise Alschuler, N.D.; James Duke, Ph.D.; Asa Hershoff, N.D., D.C.; Michael Janson, M.D.; Schuyler W. Lininger, Jr., D.C.; Patrick Quillin, Ph.D., R.D., C.N.S.; Ray Sahelian, M.D.; Alexander Schauss, Ph.D.; and Varro Tyler, Ph.D. A special thanks to Alan Gaby, M.D., for writing the foreword. This group of professionals is clearly the "cream of the crop" in the field of natural medicine.

In addition, I want to thank the many others I interviewed for this book, and those who have positively influenced my work over the years, including Carolyn DeMarco, M.D.; Kevon Arthurs, N.D.; Judy Christianson, N.D.; Herb Joiner-Bey, N.D.; Marcus Laux, N.D.; Michael T. Murray, N.D.; Steve Austin, N.D.; Joseph Pizzorno, N.D.; Zoltan Rona, M.D.; Mark Blumenthal; Siri Khalsa; and Shauna Pratt.

I am also extremely proud to be associated with the incredible people of IMPAKT Communications: Linda Selsmeyer, Creative Director; Joelle Froelich, Retail Sales Manager; Deb Michalak, Operations Manager; Janie Rosewall, Canada Division Manager; Lisa Schaal, Distribution Assistant; Jean Pigeon and Lisa Santy, Administrative Assistants; and Kelly Fisher, Graphic Designer. A special thank you to our Advertising Sales Director, Shelly Petska, for her work on this project. I would like to thank my editor and good friend, Frances FitzGerald, an incredibly talented writer, who edited this book and continues to force me into using proper grammar. A very special thanks to Kathi Magee, who is not only my sister and business partner, she is my best friend. She continues to inspire me with her strength. Also, thanks to Cody and Travis Magee, my favorite "neighbors." My gratitude and love to my biggest supporter and soulmate, Maria Dalebroux, whose patience and understanding are always appreciated.

Foreword

Nutritional and herbal therapies have a long tradition as safe and effective alternatives to conventional medicine. However, it has been only recently that natural medicine has become popular in the United States. While the public has been ahead of the medical profession in embracing these remedies, a growing number of healthcare practitioners are finally recognizing the value of "alternative" medicine. During the past ten years, an explosion of scientific research has demonstrated that many of our common chronic illnesses can be successfully prevented or treated with nutritional supplements and herbs.

However, while the potential of natural therapeutics seems almost limitless, the field in some ways is still in its infancy. Some therapies are well documented and clearly defined, but others are based largely on anecdote, opinion, or even speculation. And because natural medicine is such a new discipline in the Western healthcare system, very few guidelines and standards of care can be considered well-established. The consumer is therefore faced, in some instances, with differing "expert" opinions concerning which supplements are appropriate for which conditions, what the proper doses are, and which products are the highest quality and most effective.

If those issues are not complicated enough, we must deal with the fact that the natural products industry is not always adequately regulated. Herbs are prepared in a number of different ways and can vary greatly in potency; nutrients come in different forms and in dosages that range from therapeutic to insignificant; and the labels on supplement bottles vary in quality, from providing all of the necessary information, to being useless or even misleading. With all of these factors to consider, how is one to know which supplements to take and from whom to buy them?

In this book, Karolyn Gazella provides the reader with many of the tools needed to answer these difficult questions. Drawing on her own training in the field of natural therapeutics, plus interviews with a number of medical experts, she presents a step-by-step approach that can help us identify the highest quality products among the thousands that are on the market. *Buyer Be Wise!* discusses many important topics, including what to look for on a label, how to choose a reputable distributor, what the difference is between herbal tinctures, fluid extracts, and solid extracts, and much more. Of particular interest is the opinion of the experts concerning the risks and benefits of the most recent "wonder drugs": DHEA, melatonin, and pregnenolone.

Buyer Be Wise! is a valuable book for beginners who are entering the complicated world of nutritional and herbal supplements. It is also useful for anyone who is seeking quality and balance in the natural products they buy.

—Alan Gaby, M.D.

Dr. Gaby is the past president of the American Holistic Medical Association and the medical editor of *The Townsend Letter for Doctors*. He served on the Ad Hoc Advisory Panel of the National Institutes of Health Office of Alternative Medicine. He is the author of *Preventing and Reversing Osteoporosis* and *The Doctor's Guide to Vitamin B6*.

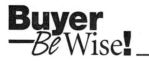

Contents

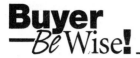

The Concept of Quality

We've all heard the saying, "One person's junk is another person's treasure." Such is the case when trying to describe quality. It's a subjective term that has become so overused, it has somehow lost some of its meaning. In some cases, defining quality is clear cut with no confusion; while at other times, the task is not so easy. To some, a quality home is simply a roof over their head, while to others, quality may take on a much more elaborate meaning.

Simply stated, quality can be described as having a high degree of superiority and excellence. Premium is another synonym. Superior value is also a great way to describe quality. No matter what description you use, the importance of quality can never be understated or overlooked. We all want quality:

- quality jobs;
- quality relationships;
- quality clothing;
- quality homes;
- and most of all, high-quality health.

You value high-quality health the most if you or a loved one has ever experienced a serious illness. It is at that time when we find out that our health is our most important asset—a gift we can either protect or take for granted. The choice is ours.

Chances are, if we are not experiencing good health, other aspects of our life suffer: our work, our relationships, and our emotional well-being.

In doing everything we can to protect the quality of our health, we search for information and incorporate healthful habits into our lives. We use all the tools available to obtain and maintain good health. During this search, we find natural medicines, concepts, and services that can help us reach our health goals. At the forefront of the natural medicine movement are nutritional supplements.

Nutritional supplements are products that contain one or more vitamin, mineral, herb, amino acid, hormone, or glandular ingredient. We know we are not alone in our enthusiasm about nutritional supplements, as sales have escalated to nearly $10 billion a year.

Unfortunately, with the countless brands and the many different types of products available, it can be difficult to know where to begin, how to determine the best value, and most of all, the highest quality. Becoming a wise consumer will help you avoid those manufacturers or distributors who are only interested in their bottom line and not your best interest.

The purpose of this book is to take away the confusion about nutritional and other natural supplements and put you in charge of your buying decisions. I have enlisted the help of some of the premier experts on natural medicine, including Marla Ahlgrimm, R.Ph.; Lise Alschuler, N.D.; James Duke, Ph.D.; Asa Hershoff, N.D., D.C.; Michael Janson, M.D.; Schuyler W. Lininger, Jr., D.C.; Patrick Quillin, Ph.D., R.D., C.N.S.; Ray Sahelian, M.D.; Alexander Schauss, Ph.D.; and Varro Tyler, Ph.D. Together, we will replace subjectivity with objectivity, providing concrete guidelines you can follow to make wise nutritional supplement buying decisions.

How important is the quality issue regarding nutritional supplements? It's **the** most important aspect. Buying an inferior product will not only waste our time and money, it could have serious negative health ramifications. After all, we are taking these supplements to either prevent illness or treat a specific condition. Not getting the results we expect and deserve will most definitely impact the quality of our health.

Fortunately, by reading this book you are taking the first important step in choosing quality products and getting the results you deserve. Congratulations!

Before you read on...

Please recognize that the purpose of this book is educational. The information provided is not intended as advice for self-diagnosis or self-treatment.

While this book focuses on nutritional supplements, it is important to keep in mind that the most successful health programs combine the best of both worlds—natural and conventional medicine. Comprehensive, integrative medicine is the way of the future. Nutritional supplements are just one part of the package. And remember, "magic bullets" do not exist. Nutritional supplements are just that, *supplements* to a healthful diet and regular exercise. Nutritional supplements, diet, exercise, and other health-promoting lifestyle activities should be used together to achieve optimum results.

This book does not mention specific product manufacturers. I am not connected with any manufacturer or distributor of nutritional products. As a research journalist and owner of a publishing company, my "product" is information. It is imperative that the information is unbiased, accurate, and reliable. The experts I have chosen to interview are also not paid royalties or commissions from product sales by any manufacturer or distributor. While some may consult with particular companies, none rely heavily on any one manufacturer for the majority of their income. I am proud of the independence that lends credibility to this book.

"The doctor of the future will give no medicine, but will interest his patient in the care of the human frame, in diet and in the cause and prevention of disease."
—Thomas Edison

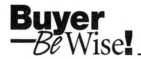

Chapter One

General Guidelines

Marketing experts often refer to the "KISS" principle—you know, "Keep It Simple Silly." When searching for quality, the KISS principle often applies. And that's good, because the more you learn about nutritional supplements, the more you will discover that this is a very complex world of unique jargon, strong philosophies, and even stronger opinions. In order to sort through the bewildering tangle of information, you need to first focus on the basics.

Here is another way of looking at the KISS principle as it relates to choosing quality nutritional supplements:

K = Keep in mind that the final decision is yours.
I = It all begins with the label.
S = Start by asking the right questions.
S = Stop focusing on price over quality.

Let's take a closer look at each of the components of this variation of the KISS principle. And the first one is the most important because it begins with you.

You are the final decision-maker. You need to make the commitment to educate yourself about your individual needs and what's available to fill those needs. This doesn't mean you have to become a natural medicine scientist. Nor do you have to spend endless hours pouring over the literature. However, it does mean you need to spend some time—as much time as you are willing to spend—learning about what you are putting into your body. Just as with the foods we eat, the nutritional supplements we take will either negatively or positively affect our health, or have no effect at all. Recognizing this is the first step toward understanding nutritional supplements. Respect your body enough to learn about the supplements you are considering. And always remember, you make the final decision based on the information you have gathered. Your doctor and the other medical experts you rely on are working for *you*—you are the boss!

The second letter of the new KISS principle is a prime example of the original KISS principle: We are going to keep things simple by focusing our attention on the label. Reading the label carefully is critical. Although this seems simple, label reading can be very challenging. In fact, many consumers today would flunk "Label Reading 101." Because this is such an important topic, it has a separate section within this chapter.

The first "S" is important because when you start by asking the right questions, chances are you will get the answers you need to make an informed buying decision. That's why this book features my interviews with a variety of natural health experts in a question-and-answer format. These are the questions you should also focus on when looking for information about a specific product, nutrient, or herb.

Remember, there are no bad questions. I am always willing to ask a question and risk looking foolish, rather than not ask it at all. So, don't be afraid to ask. My mom always told me that if you don't ask the question, you won't get an answer. I have a feeling she didn't make up that old saying; however, she got her point across.

The final "S" addresses a subject that is close to my heart: The subject of price. We need to stop focusing on price rather than quality because we all know that we get what we pay for. However, the issue of price goes much further than this. I often get frustrated when I talk to people who are disappointed in their nutritional supplement because they are not getting results. After I ask a few questions, I discover they bought, for example, a bottle of St. John's wort extract for $4.00.

In Chapter Three, "Buying Herbal Supplements," you will learn that it is physically impossible to manufacture a quality St. John's wort extract for $4.00 a bottle. When companies market these low-quality, inferior, sometimes fraudulent products, it reflects poorly on the entire natural health industry. If you buy a cheap bottle of St. John's wort and don't get results, chances are you will think poorly of the entire industry. People who are quick to say nutritional supplements don't work and are a waste of money, may be the same people who opt for the $4.00 bottle of St. John's wort rather than the $12.00 bottle. You will learn that in order to get the results you deserve, you need to look for much more than a low price.

This is such an important issue, I decided to get input from my contributing experts. My favorite response was from Varro Tyler, Ph.D., world-renowned herbal expert and author of *Honest Herbal* and *Herbs of Choice*. When I asked Dr. Tyler what he tells people who shop for price rather than quality, he said very simply, "Don't!"

Here are some other valuable comments on price:

"In general, very inexpensive products are made from poor-quality starting material. Good herbal manufacturing companies inspect and test their raw material. If the material does not meet their criteria, they will reject this material. The suppliers then sell this rejected material to other buyers who do not have quality control measures in place. These manufacturers are then able to make herbal products and sell them at a lower price because they don't pay for the quality control measures and the re-sold herbs are often sold at a lower price. Thus, a cheaper product is usually not the best quality product."
—Lise Alschuler, N.D. (see biography on page 35)

"Most of the national brands price their products within 15 to 25 percent of each other. If I see a price for something, other than a sale or promotion, that is more than 25 percent lower than the more expensive brands, I get concerned."
—Schuyler W. Lininger, Jr., D.C. (biography on page 11)

"While price should be an issue when buying nutritional supplements, I encourage people not to buy the cheapest vitamins. As in many aspects of life, you usually get what you pay for. I find poor quality supplements are often manufactured and tableted under high heat and great pressure, thus reducing the amount of nutrients available. Sometimes ingredients are added in 'token' amounts, merely to have them on the label. When looking for the best buy, look for a combination of quality manufacturing along with reasonable pricing."
—Patrick Quillin, Ph.D., R.D., C.N.S.

(biography on page 80)

"Expert formulators and production staff; scientists; research and quality control equipment; well-made and maintained equipment; safe, recyclable packaging; and pure, quality ingredients all cost companies money. But the companies that give these things priority, also give consumers the best value, because their products can be counted on for quality."
—Shauna Pratt, Canadian Marketing Consultant

Label Reading 101

All the experts I interviewed agreed: The label of the product you are buying is one of the most critical indicators of quality. You need to take the time to read and understand the label.

Unfortunately, while this sounds easy, it can also seem like learning a new language. Fortunately, there are some basic rules and recommendations to follow when evaluating the label of any nutritional supplement. Keep in mind, we will specifically discuss reading the label of an herbal product in much more detail in Chapter Three.

To begin, let's take a close look at the key components of the label. The graphic below points to the most important areas of a supplement label. Familiarize yourself with these sections of the label because they contain important information about the product you are considering.

Most of the experts interviewed for this book said label reading can be a bit "tricky" given the number of variables involved. There was a time, not too long ago, when the language of labels was as simple as learning the alphabet—vitamins A, B, C, D, and E. Today, this is not the case.

Key Label Components

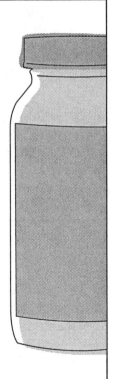

- ▶ Product Name

- ▶ Identity Statement

- ▶ Lot Number

- ▶ Expiration Date

- ▶ Ingredient Listing with Amounts

- ▶ Other Ingredients (If Any)

- ▶ Directions/Dosage

- ▶ Warnings (If Any)

- ▶ Size (Number of Tablets/Capsules)

- ▶ Manufacturer/Distributor Information

Here are some general questions you should ask yourself about the product(s) you are considering:

1. Is the product label intact, or faded or torn? "Although the design and obvious cost of a label are no guarantee of quality, they do indicate that the manufacturer is not a fly-by-night outfit. Very plain, poor-quality labels may cover a poor-quality product," explains industry consultant, Shauna Pratt.

2. Are there instructions for use, as well as warnings or contraindications (what the product should not be used with)? The more complete the label is, the better chance it is high quality.

3. Does the product have an intact, tamper-resistant seal? Remember, the tamper-resistant seal is there for a reason. Again, the outside appearance of a product is important. You will want to question the quality of the product's contents if the label and bottle are in poor condition.

4. Is there a lot number and/or an expiration date on the product you are considering? This information provides important indicators of freshness. Chances are, supplements taken past their expiration date will not harm your body, but they will rob your pocketbook because they won't be as effective. You will also need to reference the lot number if you are requesting a certificate of analysis from the manufacturer or distributor.

5. Are you familiar with the manufacturer/brand? Dealing with reputable firms with a solid reputation is very important. Find out how long the company has been in business and if you can contact them with questions or concerns.

6. Is the label comprehensive? Be sure key components are not missing. For example, ingredients without amounts (i.e., milligrams, micrograms, International Units) should be considered suspect.

For more information on label reading, I consulted with industry expert, Dr. Schuyler Lininger. Here are his recommendations on this important topic.

Ask the Expert...Dr. Schuyler Lininger

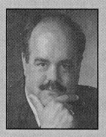 Schuyler (Skye) Lininger, D.C., is a nutritionally oriented chiropractor and publisher of *HealthNotes*, a newsletter used by over 1,000 natural food stores. He is a respected author and also heads up the most popular natural medicine on-line service.

KG—What advice do you give people for evaluating product labels?

Dr. Lininger—I tell patients to look for full ingredient disclosure. Everything should be clearly listed so it can be determined what nutrients are used and what form they are in. For example, chromium is available in several forms. The customer should be able to determine what form of chromium (i.e., picolinate, polynicotinate) is used and how many micrograms (mcg) of the actual chromium is contained in each tablet or capsule.

KG—What other things should people look for on the label?

Dr. Lininger—A full listing of excipients (inert substances), binders, fillers, and so on is important. Customers should know what things are used in the manufacturing process. It is also important that a list of things "not" included are on the label. For example, in this age of food sensitivities and allergies, the label should state if the product does "not" contain yeast, soy, lactose, dairy, and so on. Finally, an expiration or "best used before" date should be on the label, not so much for safety, but so the customer can tell if the product is fresh or old.

KG—What are some red flags consumers should watch for that could indicate poor quality?

Dr. Lininger—If the customer has never heard of the company or brand before, that's a red flag to me. Most of the well-known companies have a lot at stake in maintaining high-quality standards. It is not unusual, however, for opportunists to jump into the market with "hot" products. This happened with melatonin, DHEA, and St. John's wort. I expect it will happen again. When the well-known brands run out of stock on an unexpectedly hot product, no-name brands offer "knock-offs" that may or may not contain what the label states. I think both stores and customers should steer clear of companies they are unfamiliar with. Purchasing established and reputable brands is the surest way to ensure that the products are high quality.

So, let's review the most important aspects of reading a nutritional supplement label:
1. Be sure the product is from a quality manufacturer who is trusted, and has a reputation for high quality.
2. The label should be complete, providing a full listing of ingredients, fillers, and exact amounts, as well as warnings (if any), directions for use, and what's not in the product (yeast, dairy, etc.).
3. The label and the bottle should be neat and clean.
4. Be sure there is an expiration date on the product, and don't buy any product past its expiration.
5. Read the label carefully, paying special attention to the key ingredients.

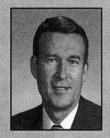
For more information on quality issues regarding nutritional supplements, I contacted respected consultant and author, Alexander G. Schauss, Ph.D.

KG—Are nutritional supplements regulated?

Dr. Schauss—Dietary supplements sold in the United States do not have to be registered with any state or federal government agency. That's right. Neither domestically produced nor imported products are registered with any government agency. Anyone can produce and/or sell a dietary supplement. As a result, efforts are increasing to self-police the industry through trade associations. It is useful for consumers to know about these efforts and how they relate to quality assurance.

KG—What action is the industry making to self-regulate nutritional supplements?

Dr. Schauss—In the United States, manufacturers can "register" products when they join the National Nutritional Foods Association (NNFA), the nation's largest natural products trade organization, which was founded in 1935. NNFA members who engage in the manufacture of dietary supplements must submit the label of every product they produce to the NNFA's Director of Science and Quality Assurance as a condition of membership. The contents of the label are entered into a computer. Periodically, the NNFA randomly tests specific supplements through independent laboratories to evaluate whether the ingredients listed on the label agree with the laboratories' analytical report. If there is a problem, the NNFA's Compliance and Label Integrity Committee notifies the manufacturer and requests immediate action. If no action is taken, the NNFA can and will make their findings public through their official trade newsletter. In addition, if the manufacturer does not resolve the problem, the manufacturer could be barred from displaying its line of products at national trade shows.

KG—How much can we depend upon the NNFA's quality assurance measures?

Dr. Schauss—Their program does not guarantee that every product you purchase from an NNFA member is what it says on the label. The program offers ethical manufacturers the opportunity of independently verifying the quality of their products. Remember, when you buy from a non-NNFA member, an independent trade organization is not policing that product. To ensure you are taking a quality product, you need to be sure the manufacturer is utilizing Good Manufacturing Practices (GMPs).

KG—What is the purpose of GMPs?

Dr. Schauss—The lack of uniform self-policing within the natural health industry resulted in the development of Congressionally mandated Good Manufacturing Practices. These are contained in a 1994 law called the Dietary Supplement Health and Education Act (DSHEA, pronounced d'shay). This requires the Food and Drug Administration (FDA) to impose uniform GMPs for the entire industry, whether they are an NNFA member or not. These Congressionally mandated and FDA-monitored GMP regulations will be in effect by the time this book is published. Any manufacturer found to be out of compliance with the government's GMPs could face legal action by the FDA. If a serious problem is uncovered, the FDA has the authority by law to shut down a manufacturer. According to the FDA, "The objective (of GMPs) is to assure that consumers are provided with safe dietary supplement products which are not adulterated or misbranded..."

KG—What exactly are GMPs?

Dr. Schauss—Basically, GMPs describe a process that must be followed in the manufacture of dietary supplements. They are modeled after good manufacturing practices for foods, not pharmaceuticals. This is because dietary supplements are much closer to foods in nature than drugs, hence require less stringent GMPs. Like foods, dietary supplements rarely cause illness or death. In fact, dietary supplements are far safer to consume than foods, causing one-sixty-thousandth as many deaths as foods each year. Nevertheless, despite an extraordinary safety record, mistakes can happen. Congress desired that if the dietary supplement industry received greater freedom to market its products without being classified as food additives or drugs, that it abide by stringent GMPs. GMPs cover every element involved in the manufacturing of dietary supplements. They include training of personnel, plant layout and sanitation facilities, equipment, warehousing, record-keeping, etc. Within each area, the manufacturer is required to maintain quality assurance and quality controls. One way consumers can find out if a product actually contains what the label says is to review the certificate of analysis.

KG—What is a certificate of analysis?

Dr. Schauss—Conscientious manufacturers of dietary supplements go out of their way to ensure that every ingredient listed is at the level indicated on the label. To make sure of this, many manufacturers send the raw materials that go into the product, as well as the finished product, to independent laboratories, which then verify and certify what the contents are.

KG—How do you know if the analysis is valid?

Dr. Schauss—Most consumers don't realize they can obtain a certificate of analysis from the manufacturer. The certificate should coincide with the lot number of the product being evaluated. Don't expect the numbers on the certificate to be in perfect agreement. Each ingredient should be slightly higher or lower than the number on the label, but within 5 to 10 percent of the label claim. If it is higher or lower than 10 percent, then there is a problem with quality control.

KG—Does it matter if the certificate was done by an independent laboratory or a manufacturer's in-house lab?

Dr. Schauss—Both certificates can be valid. Most reputable manufacturers have an in-house laboratory that monitors every facet of quality assurance and quality control. The certificate should show the name of the lab, address, and phone number. It should be dated and signed by the lab director. The lab should hold membership in a professional society. The certificate should specify that each active ingredient was tested on the raw materials and the finished product.

KG—Any final comments on this issue?

Dr. Schauss—Even if the government strictly registered and monitored every dietary supplement product in the United States, it still does not preclude the possibility that a product could reach the consumer failing to meet the claimed content on the label. One only has to look at the incidence of such problems in the pharmaceutical industry, which is much more strictly regulated, to appreciate how frequent a problem that is. For that reason, consumers need to take greater responsibility in finding out the level of quality control that goes into the dietary supplements they consume.

"Nature is doing her best each moment to make us well. She exists for no other end. Do not resist. With the least inclination to be well, we should not be sick."
—Henry David Thoreau

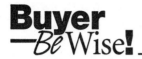

Chapter Two

Building a Strong Foundation

Any homebuilder will tell you that if you want a solid house, you need to start with a strong foundation. This is also true with nutritional supplements. There is no question that a comprehensive multivitamin/mineral supplement is the best building block possible.

What is the most commonly purchased nutritional supplement? A multivitamin/mineral formulation, of course. With total estimated supplement sales at $6 billion in the United States alone, the multi remains one of the most popular of all.

The multi's popularity is not without good reason. It's a great place to start when it comes to designing your nutritional supplement blueprint.

Why do you need a multi?

We have been led to believe that a healthful diet will provide us with all the nutrients we need to maintain optimum health. Researchers have confirmed that this is just not true. In fact, statistics tell us that more than 60 percent of us are deficient in vitamin B6, magnesium, chromium, calcium, iron, zinc, and fiber. Other common deficiencies include vitamins A, C, B1, B2, B12, and niacin. Some of these deficiencies are due to poor food choices, and some are due to the poor quality of foods themselves.

Sadly, we are a nation of overfed, undernourished individuals. And unfortunately, the "side effects" of a poor diet are deadly:

- The nation's number-one killer, heart disease, is associated with too many saturated fats and empty calories.
- High blood pressure has been linked to a diet filled with too much salt and too little potassium.
- Liver disease is associated with excessive alcohol intake.
- Too little fiber will double the chance of developing colon cancer.
- A high-fat, high-sugar diet, as well as other lifestyle factors, are involved in more than 50 percent of new cancer cases.
- Obesity, which is a key contributor to a number of serious health problems, including heart disease and high blood pressure, continues to skyrocket out of control despite an emphasis on "low-fat" eating.

Two conclusions can be made from this important information:

1. We need some dietary "insurance" if we are to protect our health and maintain optimum levels of vitality. A comprehensive multi offers that insurance.
2. Nothing can take the place of a healthful diet. "Supplements cannot make up for a deficient diet, but there are still a lot of good things a good multivitamin can offer," explains Richard N. Firshein, D.O., author and healthcare practitioner.

Surviving versus thriving

Conventional health wisdom tells us that if we meet the Recommended Dietary Allowance (RDA) of key nutrients, we will be healthy. Unfortunately, for decades, RDAs have given consumers a false sense of health security. Worse yet, most people are not getting even these marginal amounts.

"RDAs are not useful in establishing optimal health," explains Michael Janson, M.D., in his book *The Vitamin Revolution in Health Care*. "These nutrient levels are supposed to prevent deficiency diseases in most healthy people. Unfortunately, the values have been influenced by the food industry, economic considerations, and politics, not just by science."

In fact, Dr. Janson points out that while getting the RDAs for certain nutrients will help prevent the corresponding deficiency disease (i.e., vitamin C and scurvy), these levels do little to prevent degenerative diseases (heart disease, arthritis, cancer, etc.), which are at the heart of our current healthcare crisis.

"In this regard, it is not good to be average: the average American will die early of heart disease, stroke, diabetes, or cancer," concludes Dr. Janson.

In general, RDAs are ineffective dietary markers for the following reasons:

■ Nutrient requirements vary dramatically from one individual to the next. The present RDA standard only applies to healthy people who simply want to prevent deficiency, not enhance their health.

■ RDAs do not account for at-risk groups of individuals, including the elderly, women who are pregnant, lactating, or on oral contraceptives, teenagers, smokers, dieters, or people who drink alcohol or take prescription medications. Add those who are struggling with an illness, and you have a large percentage of people who need much more than the RDAs.

■ The RDAs were established more than 50 years ago, before food processing, increased sugar and fat consumption, and countless prescription and over-the-counter medications—all of which sabotage the nutrient value of our diet.

Clearly, this makes a strong case for a multi. But not just any multi will do. This is your key building block to good health, so use care when purchasing a quality multivitamin/mineral formula. With the popularity of nutritional supplements on the rise, it's not surprising that there are countless multivitamin/mineral supplements to choose from.

To help you sift through the selections, I've established some guidelines based on my research and con-
versations with a variety of healthcare professionals.

1. There is no such thing as a quality "one-a-day" multi-
   vitamin/mineral supplement. If you think you can
   take just one pill and get everything you need, you
   have been fooled by the"one-a-day"marketing cam-
   paign. Physically, it is just not possible to get all the
   minerals and vitamins you need, in the dosages you
   need, into one pill—unless, of course, the pill were
   the size of a golf ball, which would be challenging to
   swallow! Typically, you need to take at least three
   tablets each day, depending on the product.
2. Never buy a multi that does not clearly list the
   amount of each ingredient. A "laundry list" of
   ingredients without mg, IU, or mcg amounts identified is a red flag. Avoid those, because there are
   too many other good products to choose from.
3. Be sure the product does not contain potential
   allergens such as wheat, corn, milk, yeast, or fillers,
   additives, and artificial flavors or colors. "[These]
   indicate cost-cutting for profit, and in the case of
   nonfood grade fillers, such as talc and silicon, may
   lead to digestive and absorption problems,"
   according to Dr. Firshein. These substances are
   also additional, unnecessary toxins that your body
   must detoxify.
4. Stick with manufacturers who have a reputation for
   high quality. Do they make other products? Have
   other people you've talked to gotten good results
   from that specific company's products?
5. Look for a balance of important vitamins and minerals. Recognize that many of them will be in a
   higher dosage than the RDA—some, much higher.
   Although your multi can't replace a healthful diet,
   you do want it to be strong enough to provide you
   with the "nutritional insurance" you need. In my
   first book, *Help Yourself: The Beginner's Guide to
   Natural Medicine*, Judy Christianson, N.D., gave

this sound advice: "Because most people are looking for more than just the prevention of vitamin deficiency diseases, a multivitamin/mineral product that only contains 100 percent of the RDA may not be enough to support optimal health."

6. Get advice from natural health experts, books, magazines, and other quality publications, and don't be afraid to ask questions. Because a multi will become a staple in your health regimen, take time with your decision to be sure you get the most comprehensive multi. Don't shop for price, buy for quality. A cheap multi is a red flag. Remember, it costs money to make quality and not skimp on key ingredients. Even though you may pay more, it will be well worth it to get a superior multi.

7. Buy products from manufacturers and distributors who focus on education and accurate information. The information provided should be scientific, unbiased literature, not just sales information. Sometimes it can be difficult to tell what information is reliable and what is "marketing hype." There will be more about this topic in Chapter Six.

8. Choose a specialized multi (i.e., for women, men, children, seniors, etc.). "Multiples have come a long way and can give you a lot more than they used to," explains Cathy Mazur, who has been involved in the natural health industry for 20 years and owns For the Good of It, a health food store in Joliet, IL. "Technology can now provide us with multi's that are very specific to an individual's needs." A multi for a pregnant woman is completely different than a multi for a senior man. By doing a little research, you should be able to find a multi that is designed specifically for your individualized needs. "These high-tech, high-quality multi's are big sellers in our store," says Mazur.

Multivitamin/mineral supplements are available in a variety of forms: liquid, time-released, internasal, sublingual, powder, and good, old-fashioned capsules and tablets. While it has not been proven that time-released is worth the additional money, a liquid multi is often appropriate, especially for children, the elderly, or people who have difficulty swallowing capsules or tablets. Typically, tablets are used because they can "fit" more minerals in each dosage. This is very important, considering the lack of important minerals in the soil and an increase of mineral deficiencies.

In his article featured in *Natural Pharmacy*, Dr. Firshein calls the multivitamin, "king of the counter." It's a well-deserved title for an understandably popular supplement.

When developing your specific health program, begin with a strong foundation. A multivitamin/mineral supplement is the perfect building block. But don't just settle for any supplement. Do a little research and choose your supplement wisely.

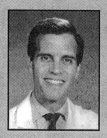
For his perspective on this topic, I consulted with Michael Janson, M.D., a respected author, radio host, and clinician. Here is his advice.

KG—How do you evaluate a quality multivitamin/ mineral supplement?

Dr. Janson—When starting a dietary supplement program, it is far easier to start with a comprehensive multivitamin/mineral combination to get all the basics. A good multi should provide high doses of all the B-complex vitamins, beta-carotene and vitamins A, E, and C, and all the minerals in RDA levels or higher except for iron, unless you have a clear need for this nutrient. Some of the minerals such as chromium and selenium have no RDA, but a good multi will have 100 to 200 mcg of each.

KG—What guidelines can people use when purchasing their multi?

Dr. Janson—A good purchasing guideline is to look at the chromium and selenium levels, and be sure the magnesium level is about 300 to 500 mg. If the brand also has about 50 mg of the main B vitamins, and contains natural vitamin E (300 to 400 IU), it is probably a good quality supplement.

Don't look for more than the basics. For example, if it contains carnitine or coenzyme Q10, they are probably not in adequate amounts to be therapeutic, but they will raise the cost.

KG—How do you respond to individuals who say supplements are unnecessary because we can get all the nutrients we need from our diet?

Dr. Janson—It is impossible to get adequate nutrients for optimal health from diet alone, especially as we age. With diet, you can prevent the basic deficiency diseases, but higher doses are essential for a high level of health and protection from environmental toxins. Commercial agriculture, early picking, transportation and storage of foods have adversely affected the nutritional quality of our groceries. Pesticides, herbicides, fungicides, and toxins in the air and water add to the burden of chemicals that we must detoxify, and extra nutrients can help. Also, with numerous health problems, dietary supplements that go beyond what our diet can supply can be therapeutic. In many cases, they can reduce or eliminate the need for medications or surgery.

KG—What is your opinion of the established Recommended Dietary Allowances (RDAs)?

Dr. Janson—The RDAs of nutrients are levels that are supposed to prevent deficiency diseases in most healthy people. Unfortunately, the values have been heavily influenced by the food industry, economic considerations, and politics, not just by science. They make the highly processed American food supply look more nutritious than it actually is.

KG—Can we use RDAs as useful measures of evaluating quality supplements?

Dr. Janson—The RDAs are not useful in establishing optimal health. You are at little risk of developing the deficiency diseases—pellagra, scurvy, or beriberi, in the overt forms, even on the standard American diet. Our modern problems are not usually deficiency diseases but degenerative diseases. Dietary supplements that go beyond what you can get from food, and at levels that are far higher than the RDA, play an important role in preventing and treating these conditions. The RDA cannot be used in evaluating the therapeutic and preventive value of large doses of dietary supplements.

I also asked Dr. Lininger what beginner's advice he gives his patients. Here are his comments:

"I often recommend a good multivitamin/mineral supplement. Sometimes tablets or capsules are not well-tolerated, so I often recommend people start with a soft-gelatin multiple that is already liquefied and easy to digest. I want to ensure the multi has at least 1,000 mg of vitamin C, 400 IU of vitamin E, 1,000 mg of calcium, 500 mg of magnesium, 10,000 IU equivalent of 'natural' beta-carotene, 200 mcg of chromium, and 200 mcg of selenium. These antioxidants and protector minerals form a solid foundation for any supplement program."

Regarding the issue of price and the multi, Dr. Quillin had this to say:

"If it seems too good to be true, i.e., much cheaper than all other comparable products, then don't buy it. I generally discourage the use of cheap multiples...While there are some poor quality nutritional supplements on the market, there are many very good products out there. Fortunately, since nutrients are relatively safe, the worst-case scenario for an unwise vitamin shopper would be wasting his or her money and delaying the potential benefits from taking good supplements."

What really is natural?

Just like the word "quality," the term "natural" conjures up all kinds of different meanings and interpretations. Some say it's been misused and abused in the "natural" health industry. However, I still feel it is a better description than "alternative," which is often used to describe the "natural" health movement.

What really is natural? This question has been hotly debated. While the dictionary has more than a dozen definitions for the word natural, for the purpose of this book, we will describe natural supplements this way:

—Natural is the opposite of synthetic, which is a substance that is synthesized or created in a laboratory to look and act like its natural counterpart. Natural nutrients are identical to the same nutrients found in foods or manufactured by the body.

One of the biggest misconceptions is that everything "natural" is good for you. In his book, *The Vitamin Revolution in Health Care*, Dr. Janson points out, "Everything natural is not necessarily healthy or beneficial to humans. For example, earthquakes, floods, and syphilis are all 'natural,' but they are not desirable."

Just because something is labeled "natural" doesn't mean you have any guarantees. You still need to carefully analyze the product.

According to the above definition, "natural" is truly

better. Natural in this sense equates to higher quality, more effectiveness, and greater benefits. In fact, many studies have shown that natural vitamins, minerals, and herbs are much better utilized by the body. That makes sense, because the body is better able to recognize and assimilate a "natural" substance than a synthetic, "manmade" substance.

For further clarification, I asked Dr. Janson about the issue of natural versus synthetic. Here is his response:

"Natural is sometimes a misleading phrase when it comes to vitamins. Most of the B vitamins in high doses are inevitably manufactured, but the molecules are exactly the same as those in foods. It is probably not possible to get all the B vitamins, and it is not necessary. On the other hand, synthetic vitamins E and D are actually different molecules than the ones naturally present in food, or in the case of vitamin D, the one that is made in the body. Synthetic beta-carotene is different from the natural carotenes. Because of these molecular differences, I recommend only the natural vitamins D and E and usually recommend the natural carotenes."

Vitamin E is a prime example of why natural is better. In laboratory studies with cancer cells, natural vitamin E significantly outperformed its synthetic counterpart. Scientists believe the synthetic component of the vitamin E actually inhibits the nutrient's ability to penetrate the cell, where it can do the most good. For this reason, natural vitamin E is preferred over synthetic. Natural forms of vitamin E include d-alpha tocopheral, d-alpha-tocopheryl acetate, and d-alpha tocopheryl succinate. The synthetic version of these has an "l" after the "d."

Pharmaceutical companies are quick to try to synthesize natural substances. A natural substance cannot be patented, which means anyone is free to market and sell the substance. But a synthesized natural substance that is slightly different than the original can then be patented and sold exclusively by the patent owner, the drug company. In fact, an estimated 30 percent of the drugs available today are derived from herbs. There is no doubt, this is big business! However, it is extremely important that you understand these synthesized sub-stances are still foreign to the body—they are not natural.

So, the lesson on "natural" is two-fold:

1. The word "natural" is not your only indication of quality. Because the term is often misused (intentionally, at times), you still need to do your homework on the product(s) you are considering. This is true for foods as well as nutritional supplements. Look for natural sources of ingredients and become familiar with terminology like d-alpha-tocopheral versus dl-alpha-tocopheral.

2. When a product is "natural," it is a better product because the body utilizes it more effectively. As you become a proficient label-reader, you will quickly recognize "unnatural" products. The general rule is to purchase natural products from a well-established manufacturer/supplier who you trust and respect.

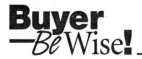

Chapter Three

Buying Herbal Supplements

Herbal supplements may be the most complex and confusing category of nutritional supplements. After all, it is here where you really *are* dealing with a foreign language as you delve into the world of European terms and Latin names. Add to this the number of different herbs and then mix in a variety of forms, and you have created a recipe that can become almost maddening.

According to *Alternative Medicine: The Definitive Guide* (Future Medicine Publishing 1993), "There are an estimated 250,000 to 500,000 plants on the earth today—the number varies depending on whether subspecies are included. Only about 5,000 of these have been extensively studied for their medicinal applications."

The enormous medicinal potential of herbal medicine cannot be denied. "Considering that 121 prescription drugs come from only 90 species of plants, and that 74 percent of these were discovered following up native folklore claims, a logical person would have to say that there may still be more jackpots out there," explains Norman R. Farnsworth, Ph.D., professor of pharmacology at the University of Illinois at Chicago.

Unfortunately, sifting through the mine field of misinformation and weeding fact from fiction can seem like a monumental task—but it can be done!

Herbal medicine provides us with an incredible realm of safe and effective healing alternatives—alternatives that consumers are demanding. "The revival of interest in herbal medicine is a worldwide phenomenon," explains Mark Blumenthal, Executive Director of the American Botanical Council.

"This renaissance is due to the growing concern of the general public about the side effects of pharmaceutical drugs, the impersonal and often demeaning experience of modern healthcare practitioners, as well as a renewed recognition of the unique medicinal value of herbal medicine," according to *Alternative Medicine: The Definitive Guide.* "In the past 150 years, chemists and pharmacists have been isolating and purifying the 'active' compounds from plants in an attempt to produce reliable pharmaceutical drugs."

Well-known examples of this include:

■ willow's bark   = aspirin
■ opium poppy   = morphine
■ foxglove   = digitalis

"The scope of herbal medicine ranges from mild-acting plant medicines to very potent ones...In between these two poles lies a wide spectrum of plant medicines with significant medical applications," explains Don Brown, N.D., noted author and expert in the field of herbal medicine. "One need only go to the United States *Pharmacopoeia* (guidelines on drugs) to see the central role that plant medicine has played in American medicine."

It's true that the power of herbal medicine cannot be questioned; however, knowing the power exists and tapping into that power are two very different things. Of course, it only makes sense that to gain the most effective benefits from herbal medicines, you must buy the right products. This concept is so simple, yet so complex.

Let's look at the different herbal forms available over-the-counter. Keep in mind, these definitions are gleaned from a variety of sources. While the descriptions are fairly clear-cut, the debate as to which form is the most effective rages on. There are no black-and-white answers, merely informed opinions.

Forms of herbal extracts

Herbal preparations are available in a variety of forms, including tinctures, fluid extracts, standardized extracts, bulk herbs, and teas. The three most controversial and most frequently compared are tinctures, fluid extracts, and standardized extracts.

■ **Tinctures.** To make a tincture, the herb is soaked in a solvent, typically alcohol and water, for a specific amount of time. The soaking can take from as little as a few hours to several days or longer. After that, the solution is pressed out and the tincture is made. Alcohol-free tinctures are made with glycerin. Typically, tinctures are considered to be more diluted and less potent than other herbal preparations. Tincture concentration is usually 1:5 or 1:10, which means that one part of herbal material is used with five or ten parts of solvent.

■ **Fluid extracts.** A fluid extract is considered more potent than a tincture. The concentration of a fluid extract is usually 1:1, which means one part of herbal material is used with every one part of solvent. Similar to tinctures, fluid extracts are made with alcohol and water, although other solvents can be used. The difference is that some of the solvent is distilled off, leading to the more highly concentrated, more potent extract.

■ **Standardized extracts.** By removing all fluid, a solid extract is created that can either be put into a capsule or tablet. Utilizing scientific techniques, an isolated compound within the plant, known to cause a therapeutic effect, is targeted. Standardization ensures each capsule has this same amount of therapeutic activity. While the entire plant is used, the same degree of the isolated active component is maintained. Many experts believe this form of extract provides the most potent, consistent therapeutic benefits.

When addressing the question of which form of herbal medicine is most effective, Dr. Donald Brown explained in his book, *Herbal Prescriptions for Better Health* (Prima 1996):

"This is another question without a clear-cut answer. Herbal medicines come in many forms. You may have garlic, ginger, or turmeric with your meals. You may choose to have some chamomile tea for your upset stomach. Goldenseal tincture will probably soothe your sore throat better than a capsule. A concentrated extract of ginkgo in tablet form, however, will be far more effective than a tincture in treating poor circulation."

To further understand these forms, it is important to clarify the difference between concentration versus potency:

■ Concentration means the amount of herb used compared to the amount of solvent. Obviously, a 1:1 concentration will be more powerful than a 1:10 concentration, which has more solvent compared to herbal material—10 times more solvent, to be exact.

■ Potency can be more appropriately applied to the degree of active constituents within a particular herb, which relates to standardization. This is different than concentration. Many experts believe that because standardized extracts have consistent potency, they provide a more consistent, accurate dosage.

So, as you can see, when it comes to buying herbal supplements, there are many options and much to learn. Because this issue is so important and complex, I have enlisted the help of three highly respected herbal experts and recognized authorities on the topic of plant medicines: Varro Tyler, Ph.D., retired professor from Purdue University; James Duke, Ph.D., retired ethno-botanist with the USDA; and Lise Alschuler, N.D., practicing naturopathic physician and educator.

HERBAL EXPERTS

Ask the Expert...Dr. Varro Tyler

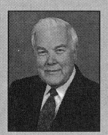
Varro Tyler, Ph.D., Sc.D., is a retired distinguished professor from Purdue University, where he spent 20 years on the faculty. He is a graduate of the University of Nebraska and did graduate work at Yale and the University of Connecticut. Dr. Tyler is a respected author and lecturer.

Ask the Expert...Dr. James Duke

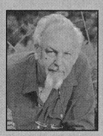
James Duke, Ph.D., spent 30 years as a botanist and ecology researcher for the USDA, and has lived among the natives in the world's rainforests. A highly respected herbal educator, Dr. Duke's latest book is *The Green Pharmacy*.

Ask the Expert...Dr. Lise Alschuler

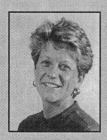
Lise Alschuler, N.D., is a practicing naturopathic physician and educator. She graduated from Bastyr University in 1994. Currently, she is chair of the Botanical Medicine Department of Bastyr University. She teaches naturopathic medical students and has a private practice.

Dr. Varro Tyler

KG—Dr. Tyler, why are you a strong proponent of standardized herbal extracts?

Dr. Tyler—You can't just grind up an herb into a powder and put it in a capsule. There's just too much variation that occurs in nature. The only sensible solution to get uniformity of these herbs is standardization. I've seen some rather tricky labels lately where the manufacturer has said standardized to contain 125 mg per capsule. That isn't what standardization is. Standardization is not the amount in the capsule; it is the potency of the active constituent. You have to read the labels very carefully.

KG—How do we know we're getting what we pay for?

Dr. Tyler—You need to find a reliable company. Standardized extracts from a reliable company is just about the only thing you have to go by. The problem is, we have companies that have excellent products, but then there are those who use hyperbolic exaggeration of claims and make inferior products. That gives everyone in the field a kind of snake-oil reputation.

KG—What advice do you give people who want to start buying and taking herbal products?

Dr. Tyler—Look first for the common names of the herb in the heading of the label. The second thing to look for on the label is the active components of the product and the specific standardized percentage amount. It is difficult for the typical layperson to sort out the facts from fiction. People should try to get as much reliable, independent information as possible to educate themselves on this subject.

Dr. James Duke

KG—What influences the quality of herbal products?

Dr. Duke—So many factors play a part in the quality of an herb. Some factors over which we don't have a lot of control are growing, soil, and weather conditions. Other factors such as drying conditions, handling, and storage, play a very important part in the final analysis and can be controlled. You don't create quality; you only preserve it. A manufacturer can't make the herb any better, stronger, more potent, etc. than what Nature provides. A good manufacturer can, however, amplify the good and diminish the bad via processing. But a bad manufacturer can mess it up in the handling and processing, thereby allowing the natural active (i.e., therapeutic) properties of the plant to deteriorate.

KG—What forms of herbal medicines are best?

Dr. Duke—Different strokes for different folks. Different processes for different end results. I favor tinctures when dealing with herbs whose activities depend largely on their aromatic constituents. For culinary herbs and refreshing herb teas, I prefer the unstandardized herb, fresh from my unpampered but organic back yard, nurtured, watched like a baby, and harvested personally by yours truly. Conversely, I almost never harvest my medicinals...The quality product in the capsule is clean, easy, efficient, and relatively economical. With echinacea, I sometimes take both tincture and capsule when the flu is going around, knowing that the capsule contains more of some active ingredients than the tinctures and vice versa.

KG—What is your opinion of standardized extracts?

Dr. Duke—Standardized extracts allow the active ingredient to be measured. Before I started compiling my database more than a decade ago, I wasn't keen on standardization. But as I compiled, I saw horrendous quantitative variations in the active biochemicals, usually ten-fold, sometimes a hundred or a thousand-fold. I became convinced that standardization was worth the effort and cost involved. Accurate measurement of active constituents allows the herbal extract to be duplicated again and again, assuring consistent potency in every batch...It also assures the consumer of consistent levels of active ingredients in each dose. Also, dried standardized extracts can deliver higher amounts of certain active ingredients. Liquid extracts, however, may have the advantage of entering the bloodstream a bit faster, and for some are easier to take than capsules or tablets.

KG—What advice do you give people on reading the label of an herbal product?

Dr. Duke—If it is standardized, you are in general getting a more reliable product than one whose label does not indicate standardization. The label should tell you what the major active ingredients are and if any preservatives are added (such as natural antioxidants and other preservatives). Modern labels should also tell you how much to take. If there is only a common name (and not the Latin name) and you've never heard of it, don't buy it. Some unscrupulous dealers intentionally use obscure or contrived names. Consumers should look for a stated amount of extract (xx mg per capsule) along with a stated quantity of active ingredients (standardized for xx mg of xxxxx).

KG—Does concentration provide any indication of quality?

Dr. Duke—Many extracts state a ratio of 4:1 or 50:1, which means that 4 or 50 pounds of a product went in and one pound came out. While this shows that a product is concentrated, it is simply a recipe. If the label doesn't state what and how much of an active ingredient is contained in the product, then there is still a very real possibility that the product may not contain any, or enough of, the active ingredient to be of benefit. Remember, 50 pounds of a low-quality herb simply produces one pound of a low-quality, inactive herbal concentrate.

KG—What advice do you give people who want to shop for herbs based on price?

Dr. Duke—Compare dosages. Sometimes the cheapest product requires two to three capsules to equal one capsule of another brand. If one brand is substantially less than the other brands, it is often, though not invariably, a good indication that quality has been compromised. If price is the only criteria, it is possible that some products may be O.K. and produce the necessary results, while the next batch of the very same product(s) may be substandard and you won't get the same results. Consumers should remember that they are putting these products in their bodies and looking for consistent therapeutic results.

KG—Any final words of advice?

Dr. Duke—Be sure the label lists all contents, including any contraindications and when to take the product. Be sure the herb is properly identified with the scientific name for those herbs that don't have well-recognized common names. Read labels very carefully and know what you are getting in each capsule. If the product says it will cure everything, look for another product.

Dr. Lise Alschuler

KG—What are some of the key advantages of tinctures and fluid extracts?

Dr. Alschuler—Although fluid extracts are more concentrated, tinctures and fluid extracts are very similar. I will talk about them as one, referring to them as tinctures. In general, I find most tinctures to be effective and reliable. Alcohol is an excellent extracting agent and preservative. Tinctures are also easily absorbed and clinically effective. Tinctures can be easily mixed together, which allows for individual formulations.

KG—Are there disadvantages of tinctures?

Dr. Alschuler—Some individuals cannot tolerate alcohol or the taste of tinctures. Tinctures of some plants may be too weak to generate pharmacological effects. Tinctures are expensive relative to teas or to some standardized extracts. It is uncommon to find tinctures that are standardized. Therefore, it can be difficult to obtain consistent dosing and effects.

KG—What is your opinion of standardized extracts?

Dr. Alschuler—Standardized extracts contain standard concentrations of constituents. Therefore, it is possible to pharmacologically dose the plant extract in a consistent, reliable fashion. The capsule or tablet form of standardized extracts is well-tolerated by most individuals. The extraction methodology allows for significant concentration of the plant. For instance, a strong tincture is a 1:2 concentration. A typical standardized extract may be equivalent to 20:1. Standardized extracts also have a long shelf life if properly stored.

KG—Are there any disadvantages of standardized extracts?

Dr. Alschuler—The herbs in standardized extracts must be dried first in order to be made into standardized extracts. The herbs must be powdered first, which increases the oxidation of certain constituents. This can alter the composition and biochemical effect of the plant. The water content of the plant is distilled off, and thus the subtle or vital energetic effects of the plant are not evident. Capsules and tablets also require fillers and binding agents, which can be detrimental to health, and some individuals may be allergic to them.

KG—Do you consider alcohol-free tinctures to be effective?

Dr. Alschuler—I have not had as good results with alcohol-free tinctures as I have had with tinctures. They are just not as effective. Glycerin, which is used in place of alcohol, is a poor extractor and does not effectively separate the plant material.

KG—What are some red flags to watch out for that indicate poor quality of an herbal product?

Dr. Alschuler—Incomplete labeling of the product is a red flag. In addition, unfortunately, there are many products on the market that contain cosmetic ingredients. In other words, the product contains herbs in order to appear as a complete product. In reality, some or all of the herbs are in amounts far below their range of therapeutic efficacy.

KG—What is your opinion of products that contain many different herbal extracts?

Dr. Alschuler—In general, only one to three unstandardized herbs will fit into a standard-size capsule in order to reach their therapeutic dosage ranges, assuming a daily dose of three to six capsules. With standardized herbs, one to perhaps four herbs will fit into a capsule and approximate their daily therapeutic dosages.

KG—Do you have any other final words of advice?

Dr. Alschuler—The herbal extract should taste like the herb. If a tincture just tastes like alcohol or diluted water, it is probably not good. Herbal tinctures always have a taste and aroma and often a color characteristic to the plant. It is possible to become familiar with these qualities for the different plant extracts and then utilize this information as a basis of comparison. Powdered herbs, even standardized extracts, should also have a taste characteristic to the plant. If a powdered herbal extract doesn't taste like anything, it is probably a poor-quality extraction and will not be very effective. In addition, if consumers are in doubt as to the quality of an herbal extract, they should obtain expert advice from a naturopathic doctor or a healthcare professional trained in herbal medicine.

It is obvious that no matter what form of an herb you are buying, certain aspects must be consistent to ensure quality:

- Look for a descriptive label that outlines exactly what is in the product, how much, and how to take it.
- Buy reputable brands from manufacturers who have a history of marketing herbal products. These manufacturers have much to lose if they begin skimping on quality.
- Trial and error may be necessary with the different forms to discover which form best suits your needs. Remember, the form may vary, based on what you are trying to accomplish at the time. To alleviate symptoms of an illness or treat a specific condition, a standardized extract will be more powerful. As a preventive, or in combination with other treatments, a tincture or fluid extract may be appropriate. As Dr. Duke explained, he sometimes uses both the tincture and capsule of echinacea when he feels the flu coming.
- Educate yourself as much as possible about specific herbal product(s) you are considering. Rely on books, magazines, and educational literature that are not tied to any one manufacturer. This will provide you with an accurate, unbiased perspective.

QUICK REFERENCE GUIDE TO COMMON HERBAL MEDICINES

Herb	**Key Use(s)**

■ **Bilberry** — Eye Health
Night vision; diabetic retinopathy; macular degeneration; cataracts; glaucoma; varicose veins

■ **Cayenne** — Varied
Atherosclerosis (clogged arteries); pain disorders; cluster headaches; arthritis; psoriasis

■ **Echinacea** — Immune System
Colds and flu; infections; candida/yeast infections; cancer

■ **Feverfew** — Migraines
Migraine headache; fever; inflammation

■ **Garlic** — Heart/Immunity
High cholesterol levels; high blood pressure; circulation; colds and flu; candida/yeast infections; cancer; diabetes; infection

■ **Ginger** — Motion Sickness
Nausea and vomiting; motion sickness; arthritis; migraine headache; digestion

■ **Ginkgo biloba** — Brain Function
Memory loss associated with aging; early stage Alzheimer's; poor circulation; ringing in the ears; depression; impotence

■ **Goldenseal** — Immune System
Infections (antibiotic activity); cancer

Herb	**Key Use(s)**

■ **Hawthorn**   Heart Function
*Angina (heart spasms); atherosclerosis;
congestive heart failure; high blood pressure*

■ **Grape seed**   Heart/Immunity
*Atherosclerosis; diabetes; varicose veins; wound
healing; macular degeneration; diabetic retinopathy;
immune stimulation*

■ **Green tea**   Immune System
Cancer prevention

■ **Kava**   Anxiety
Anxiety; depression; insomnia

■ **Milk Thistle**   Liver Health
*Liver disorders; liver protection; hepatitis;
cirrhorsis; gallstones; psoriasis*

■ **Peppermint**   Irritable Bowel
*Irritable bowel syndrome (IBS); gallstones;
gastrointestinal tract (GI) disorders*

■ **St. John's wort**   Depression
Mild to moderate depression

■ **Saw palmetto**   Prostate Health
*Enlarged prostate, also known as benign
prostatic hyperplasia (BPH)*

■ **Valerian**   Insomnia
Insomnia; stress and anxiety

Sources: *Herbs of Choice* by Varro E. Tyler, Ph.D. (Pharmaceutical Products Press, 1994);
Herbal Prescriptions for Better Health by Don Brown, N.D. (Prima, 1996);
The Healing Power of Herbs by Michael T. Murray, N.D. (Prima, 1995)

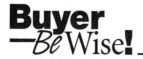

Chapter Four

Buying Hormone Supplements

Hormone supplements are the latest "craze" in the natural health industry. First there was DHEA, then melatonin, then pregnenolone. And let's not forget about progesterone. They are all available over-the-counter and are getting plenty of media attention.

We've read the headlines and heard the claims:

"The new fountain of youth"

"Increase energy"

"Enhance your sex drive"

"Elevate your mood"

"Stimulate the immune system, reduce stress, and yes, you can even alleviate the symptoms of PMS, menopause, and arthritis."

Can this be true? Are these hormones really the panacea the press is pushing? Or, are these exaggerated statements simply designed to sell more product? The answer, quite frankly, is yes and no.

Yes...

—much of the excitement is warranted as people report a variety of impressive benefits.

—evidence suggests that hormones can, in fact, slow the aging process and help reduce the risk of disease.

No...

—they are not magic bullets or cure-alls.

—they are not appropriate for everyone.

Two of the most important questions about hormones are: 1. Are they safe? and 2. Who should take them?

To answer these questions thoroughly, we need to understand these popular natural medicines.

Hormones defined

Hormones are critical to our existence. They are substances produced in the body that regulate our development on many different levels. Hormones help create who we are, how we think, feel, and respond to each other.

Hormones are created in our endocrine glands: pituitary, thyroid, parathyroids, pancreas, adrenals, ovaries, testes, pineal, and thymus glands. To a lesser degree, they are also made in the stomach, small intestines, liver, kidneys, and brain. Once they are created, they circulate through the bloodstream, regulating tissue and organ function throughout the body.

"Our hormonal systems maintain a delicate metabolic balance throughout the body," explains Joseph Pizzorno, N.D., president of Bastyr University, in his book, *Total Wellness* (Prima, 1996). "Both under- and over-activity of any of the hormonal systems can cause widespread dysfunction."

This is why natural hormone supplements may actually have a positive effect on preventing or even reversing the aging process. However, let's keep in mind that these substances are very different than other nutritional supplements. There are complex interactions between the hormones and their influence on a variety of body functions.

In order for hormones to do their job, they must connect with a receptor, just like a key fits into a lock. "Once the hormone binds with its receptor, it is transported into the nucleus, or message center of the cell, where the message is received and the hormone can begin doing its job," explains registered pharmacist Marla Ahlgrimm, R.Ph., in her booklet, *Hormone Replacement: An Individualized*

Approach to Restoring Balance. "While it sounds like a lengthy process, it is carried out hundreds of times around the clock, every day. In the myriad of chemicals, nutrients, cells, and substances in our bodies, hormones are the sparks that make things happen."

Let's first provide a general description of each of the hormones presently available over-the-counter as nutritional supplements or creams. We will discuss possible side effects and contraindications in more detail with hormone expert Ray Sahelian, M.D.

Melatonin. The first hormone to hit the natural health scene was melatonin, commonly called nature's sleeping pill. Every night, the pineal gland in the brain manufactures melatonin to help us sleep. Originally thought of as a cure for jet lag, research is now showing that melatonin may have many other important health-promoting benefits. Because it is a powerful antioxidant, it can stimulate the immune system. This is where the anti-aging claims/benefits stem from. In addition, research has indicated melatonin may show promise in the treatment of cancer because it enhances the immune system. It may also lower cholesterol levels, which benefits the cardiovascular system. By helping to alleviate our number one and two deadliest diseases, it's no wonder this hormone is being touted as an anti-aging "wonder drug."

As we age, we produce less melatonin, which can result in insomnia and a weakened immune system. The idea is that melatonin supplementation can essentially fool the body into believing it is still young.

Here is what Dr. Patrick Quillin wrote about melatonin in *Health Counselor* magazine: "Melatonin is the master clock in the body. Animal studies have found a 17 percent increase in life span with supplements of melatonin."

DHEA. Fortunately, dehydroepiandrosterone is most commonly referred to by its abbreviation—DHEA. This hormone is manufactured in the adrenal glands of both men and women. The adrenal glands are located just above the kidneys. Of the more than 150 different hormones made in the adrenals, DHEA is the most abundant.

The adrenal glands regulate the stress response in the body. High stress levels can weaken the adrenal glands. Conversely, weakened adrenal glands will negatively influence how we respond to stress. Adrenal exhaustion (i.e., high stress) can lead to poor health.

As with melatonin, DHEA levels decline as we age. Research has shown that DHEA can positively influence the immune system, possibly lower blood cholesterol levels, improve insulin function, and help with weight loss. Specific conditions that may benefit from DHEA include lupus, rheumatoid arthritis, multiple sclerosis, diabetes, and osteoporosis. Animal studies have even shown DHEA to be effective in decreasing the incidence of a variety of cancers.

Because DHEA gets converted into estrogen (as well as other hormones), DHEA can have a positive effect on menopause. In fact, a recently published human study on DHEA evaluated its effect on postmenopausal women. One of the outcomes of DHEA supplementation was a significant increase in bone density, which is a key concern of menopausal women. An estimated 24 million Americans suffer from osteoporosis, a potentially crippling condition.

Highly respected medical doctor and researcher Alan Gaby has said DHEA "...may turn out to be the most important medical advancement of the past decade."

"As time goes by, more and more research will be done on the effects of DHEA; however, for the time being, what we know is very encouraging," says physician and medical writer Ray Sahelian, M.D. Dr. Sahelian has written cutting-edge books on melatonin, DHEA, pregnenolone, and other natural compounds.

Pregnenolone. While pregnenolone (preg) is also made in the adrenal glands, it is produced in the liver, skin, and ovaries as well. The brain can also use cholesterol to make pregnenolone. Enzymes in the body help convert cholesterol to preg. It is manufactured in varying amounts in different parts of the body. Preg can be converted to progesterone, which can then be turned into cortisol (another important adrenal hormone). Preg can also be converted to DHEA, which can then be made into testosterone or estrogens. It all depends on what the body needs. As with the other hormones, the pituitary gland (located in the brain) controls and regulates the amount of preg released into the body.

"There's always interaction and communication between the pituitary gland and the rest of the organs in our body," explains Dr. Sahelian. "When the production of hormones in the adrenal glands is too high, the pituitary gland sends signals to reduce production. When the amounts of adrenal hormones made are too low, the pituitary gland again sends signals, this time to stimulate further production. There's always a balance to be maintained."

As with the other hormones, preg declines as we age. According to Dr. Sahelian, about 60 percent less preg is made at age 75 compared to age 35. As expected, a variety of conditions may benefit from this hormone. It is believed to play an important role in memory, mood, energy levels, PMS, menopause, and immunity. Unfortunately, there are few formal human studies with preg.

"A review of Medline, the computer system that records all articles published in scientific journals, shows only a few studies published on preg in 1995 and 1996, and only a couple involve human subjects," writes Dr. Sahelian in his booklet on preg. "…our knowledge about preg, at least in the near future, will mostly come from individuals using this hormone and the clinical experience of physicians prescribing preg to their patients."

Progesterone. The hormone that has been available over-the-counter for the longest period of time is progesterone. This hormone is manufactured in the ovaries in women and in small amounts in the testes of men. The adrenal glands in both men and women also produce some progesterone. As mentioned previously, progesterone is made from pregnenolone.

Progesterone serves many important functions. One of the most important ones involves the female reproductive cycle. "Pregnancy would not be possible without progesterone," says registered pharmacist and women's health expert Marla Ahlgrimm, R.Ph. "Progesterone prepares the lining of the uterus for the implantation of the fertilized egg. It then helps maintain it during pregnancy."

Key conditions progesterone can help include osteoporosis, menopause, and premenstrual syndrome (PMS). Leading women's health expert Christiane Northrup, M.D., has this to say about progesterone:

"Natural progesterone, in combination with lifestyle changes, often produces profound improvement in PMS symptoms. In their capacity as neurotransmitters, estrogen and progesterone clearly affect mood. Estrogen, if unopposed by progesterone, tends to irritate the nervous system. Progesterone, on the other hand, is associated with tranquility."

Because of its far-reaching benefits, many experts believe progesterone is even more important to the body, especially the female body, than estrogen. Dr. Alan Gaby has said in his book, *Preventing and Reversing Osteoporosis* (Prima, 1994) that progesterone "could turn out to be the most important breakthrough in decades in relation to osteoporosis treatment and prevention...Twenty years from now, scientists may look back and wonder why we focused so much on estrogen, while virtually ignoring progesterone. The use of progesterone may eliminate the need for estrogen replacement therapy in many cases."

Dr. Northrup explains that progesterone usage helps restore the important balance between estrogen and progesterone, two key hormones for female health.

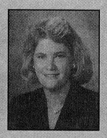
To learn more about progesterone, I consulted with Marla Ahlgrimm, co-founder of Madison Pharmacy Associates, Inc., the nation's first pharmacy specializing in women's health and natural hormone replacement.

KG—Who would be a good candidate for progesterone supplementation?

MA—Women with fertility problems, post-partum depression, PMS, perimenopause, and menopause may all benefit from the use of natural progesterone. In each of these cases, I recommend a natural progesterone cream.

KG—Why is the cream form of progesterone the best way to supplement?

MA—Progesterone cream offers distinct advantages. First, when applied this way, the hormone is quickly and easily absorbed. When a hormone is taken through the skin, it bypasses the liver and begins to course directly through your bloodstream. In addition, you can use small dosages to relieve symptoms. Cream is also more appealing to women who dislike taking medication orally.

KG—What about wild yam creams? Do they provide the same benefits as natural progesterone creams?

MA—Some manufacturers advertise that their progesterone products are derived from wild yams or contain wild yam extract. While these creams may be good products, they really have nothing to do with natural progesterone. Wild yam does not contain progesterone and your body does not convert wild yam extract into progesterone. In addition, creams that contain natural progesterone have progesterone USP, a pharmaceutical-grade product, added to them.

KG—If these products contain pharmaceutical-grade progesterone, how can they be called natural?

MA—Because this form of progesterone is bioidentical, meaning the molecule is the same as the progesterone naturally manufactured by the body. Therefore, it is completely "natural" to the human body. Synthetic progestins, like Provera, are not bioidentical and "natural" to the human body. That's why we often see more side effects with these conventionally used progestins.

KG—How can a woman be sure she is purchasing a quality progesterone cream?

MA—This is difficult. A 1995 study by Aeron Labs found that of the 27 different creams tested, 12 contained more than 400 mg of progesterone per ounce, which is the amount required for a therapeutic or medicinal effect. In contrast, five of the creams contained between 2 and 15 mg per ounce, and 10 creams contained less than 2 mg or no progesterone per ounce at all. Many manufacturers are vague when asked exactly how much progesterone is added to their product. If you can't easily ascertain this information, it's best to look for another product. Also, let your results be your guide.

KG—How does a woman know if she needs progesterone or if her progesterone cream is working?

MA—Whether a prescription or over-the-counter progesterone cream is used, I recommend hormone levels be tested before using the medication. Saliva testing is a reliable, accurate, and convenient way to evaluate the hormones you have circulating in your body. Continued monitoring of hormone levels is also important.

Ask the Expert...Ray Sahelian, M.D.

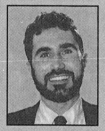

Dr. Ray Sahelian obtained a bachelor of science degree in nutrition from Drexel University and completed his doctoral training at Thomas Jefferson Medical School. He is a respected physician, medical writer, and lecturer.

To get information on melatonin, DHEA, and pregnenolone, I contacted best-selling author on the subject of hormones, Ray Sahelian, M.D. I work with Dr. Sahelian on a regular basis as he is the medical editorial consultant for our *Nature's Impact* magazine and *The American Journal of Natural Medicine*. In addition, we have published a series of informational booklets by Dr. Sahelian. For more information on Dr. Sahelian, visit his web site at www.raysahelian.com.

KG—In general, when your patients want to take an over-the-counter hormone, what advice do you give them?

Dr. Sahelian—Hormones are not as simple to self-administer as are nutrients such as vitamin C. The research on these over-the-counter hormones is still relatively new. Before embarking on a long-term replacement therapy program, read a book about these hormones that presents the information in a non-biased way. The book or article should present both the positive and negative aspects of taking these hormones. I also recommend supervision by a health-care practitioner when supplementing with these hormones.

KG—What label-reading advice do you give people?

Dr. Sahelian—Read the label carefully to make sure you know exactly how much of the hormone is present in one tablet or capsule. Read to see what time of the day to take it. In general, DHEA and pregnenolone are best taken in the morning, while melatonin is taken in the evening. As for DHEA, some products contain yam extracts and claim this converts to DHEA in the body. The human body does not have the ability to convert yam extracts into DHEA. The product you buy should say it contains actual DHEA on the label. Buy the lowest dosage available. As for melatonin, this would be 0.3 or 0.5 mg. DHEA and pregnenolone should not be sold over-the-counter in a dose greater than 5 or 10 mg.

KG—Are there groups of people who should never take any kind of over-the-counter hormone?

Dr. Sahelian—Those who are pregnant, have thyroid abnormalities or other endocrine problems, have heart irregularities, or are on medicines should always consult their physician before taking hormones.

KG—Out of all of the hormones available over-the-counter, is there one that is more "dangerous" than the others?

Dr. Sahelian—DHEA and pregnenolone in high dosages, such as 30 mg or more, can cause heart irregularities in susceptible individuals.

KG—What advice do you give about the long-term use of these over-the-counter hormones?

Dr. Sahelian—Many people benefit tremendously from hormones, including improvements in brain function, memory, mood, energy levels, sexual drive, immune system, and a reduction in arthritis symptoms. However, long-term use in high dosages, greater than 10 mg, is currently discouraged until more information is available. I recommend "hormone holidays." This means going off these hormones once in a while. I suggest a week off every two weeks.

Now, let's get Dr. Sahelian's perspective on the individual hormones themselves, beginning with melatonin.

KG—Is melatonin addictive, like many prescription insomnia drugs?

Dr. Sahelian—Since no studies in humans have yet been published specifically addressing this question, I can't make a definitive statement about melatonin's addictive potential. I can only state my own experience and the experience of my patients, who feel that melatonin is not physically addictive. However, it can be habit-forming in some people.

KG—Are there any withdrawal symptoms if you stop taking melatonin?

Dr. Sahelian—Data from my surveys suggest that withdrawal symptoms from the abrupt discontinuation of short-term melatonin use are uncommon. It's still too early to tell whether suddenly stopping melatonin after a few years of regular, nightly use will lead to withdrawal symptoms. However, the "hormone holidays" discussed earlier should help alleviate this problem. I recommend, at most, melatonin to be taken every other night; preferably, every third night.

KG—Based on your extensive research, do you feel melatonin is a safe supplement to take?

Dr. Sahelian—Since melatonin is produced naturally, the body has evolved mechanisms to remove excessive amounts. It is metabolized by the liver and possibly other organs. No reports of any serious side effects have yet been reported in the medical literature. Of course, no substance on this planet can be guaranteed to be 100 percent safe. However, based on the available clinical and scientific data thus far, I believe there is enough evidence to support the occasional use of melatonin. It is a good alternative to prescription sleeping pills. Begin with very low doses, such as 0.2 mg. Adjust upwards the following night if that dose is not effective.

KG—What are some of the side effects that can occur when using melatonin supplements?

Dr. Sahelian—Side effects usually only occur with doses greater than 1 mg. They can include:

- Morning grogginess or fuzzy thinking.
- Tiredness or sleepiness the next day.
- Waking up in the middle of the night and not being able to get back to sleep.
- Worse sleep than normal.
- Headaches or depressed feelings.

All these side effects are indications that the dosage may be too high. More infrequent side effects reported are bad dreams or nightmares, and lower sex drive. On very rare occasions, mild stomach upset or nausea, dizziness or light-headedness, diarrhea, constipation, and itchiness have been reported.

KG—How can we be assured we are buying an effective melatonin product?

Dr. Sahelian—Since the FDA does not regulate melatonin, its purity cannot be guaranteed. In 1996, however, the NNFA did an evaluation of 42 melatonin products and found 38 to be accurate to the label. My hope is that as the popularity of melatonin increases, organizations engaged in consumer protection will choose to analyze and certify the purity and content of melatonin from different manufacturers and distributors. This certification would ease the concerns of many who wish to use melatonin regularly but are worried about possible impurities or inaccurate labeling.

KG—Let's switch gears now and discuss DHEA. What are the side effects that can occur with the use of DHEA?

Dr. Sahelian—Every medicine has its ideal dosage. Too little is ineffective, and too much can be counterproductive. This is also true for DHEA. Excessive doses of DHEA can lead to side effects such as acne, irritability, overstimulation, insomnia, and headaches. Occasionally, too much DHEA can trigger hair growth in women in unwanted places, such as the face, and hair loss can occur on the scalp. Some sensitive individuals get side effects on as low a dose as 5 mg. There have been infrequent reports of heart irregularities in those who have taken a large dose at one time, such as 50 or 100 mg. Even a dose of 25 mg has induced heart palpitations in those with weak hearts. I recommend low dosages of DHEA, such as 2 to 10 mg, to those who are interested in trying this hormone over-the-counter.

KG—In general, do you feel DHEA is safe?

Dr. Sahelian—I have interviewed several researchers and clinicians who are familiar with DHEA. Their combined experience with thousands of patients indicates that DHEA has few side effects when used appropriately and in low doses. Nonetheless, it is still best that we proceed cautiously until more long-term studies are available. DHEA, in my opinion, can be unsafe in certain sensitive individuals in dosages greater than 15 mg.

KG—What about contraindications? Does DHEA interact negatively with any drugs?

Dr. Sahelian—Unfortunately, there are hardly any studies published on the combination of DHEA with prescription or non-prescription drugs. However, based on what is known about DHEA and my knowledge of medicines, I can provide some tentative suggestions. Keep in mind, it is a good idea to consult with your physician about the appropriateness of taking any medications in combination.

■ **Anti-depressants.** Because DHEA can elevate mood in some individuals, anti-depressant medicine dosages may be reduced.

■ **Estrogen.** Since DHEA gets converted to estrogen, hormone replacement therapy dosages may have to be altered.

■ **Aspirin and blood thinners.** DHEA can act as a mild blood thinner, so dosages can be affected.

■ **Stimulants.** Because DHEA is also a stimulant, it is not a good idea to combine high doses of this hormone with other stimulants.

■ **Insulin.** There are no apparent interactions that we know of. It's probably fine to use a low dose of DHEA if you have diabetes.

■ **Thyroid hormones.** The combination of DHEA and thyroid hormones can lead to overstimulation. Caution is indicated.

KG—When is the best time to take DHEA?

Dr. Sahelian—The adrenal glands make lots of DHEA in the early morning, and production drops dramatically throughout the day. It is best to take DHEA in the morning to act in concert with this natural daily pattern. A high evening dose has been shown to cause insomnia in some individuals.

KG—At what age should a person begin thinking about DHEA supplements?

Dr. Sahelian—Most physicians who incorporate DHEA replacement therapy in their practice will test people starting in their 40s.

KG—Now let's address pregnenolone. Do you believe this hormone is safe?

Dr. Sahelian—Preg has the potential to benefit many individuals when used appropriately. Unfortunately, there's still a lot to be learned about this fascinating hormone. In both animal and human studies, preg has been shown to be safe. Common side effects reported while taking high doses of preg include irritability, headaches, and insomnia and acne. As with DHEA, high dosages can cause heart palpitations.

KG—What is the appropriate dosage of preg?

Dr. Sahelian—Research with preg is more limited than that of DHEA. I recommend that people be supervised by a healthcare professional and start with 10 mg or 5 mg if sensitive to medicines. If, after a few days, the person does not notice a sense of well-being, then the dose can be increased to 20 mg. Preg can accumulate in the body, especially in the central nervous system, so be patient.

Once people start noticing the effects, they can cut back their dosage. Some people do well on a maintenance of just 2 to 5 mg per day.

KG—Because preg levels drop as we age, like DHEA and melatonin, does this make it more appropriate for people over age 40?
Dr. Sahelian—Yes. Individuals in their 20s and 30s can use preg, but only temporarily and only for a specific medical condition, such as PMS.

KG—In general, do you find there is a huge quality problem with these hormone supplements?
Dr. Sahelian—Yes and no. A chemist friend of mine did an informal test of some melatonin products on the market. He found one, a pineal gland extract, that did not contain melatonin at all. On the other hand, a number of DHEA products tested at our Longevity Research Center were found to be accurate as far as their claims on the label. All of the 14 different products tested contained within 90 to 100 percent of what was claimed on the bottle. You can see the results of that analysis at our web site, www.raysahelian.com.

To summarize...

The topic of natural hormone supplements is complicated, controversial, and fascinating. As Dr. Sahelian said, supplementing with hormones is not as simple as supplementing with vitamins. These are complex molecules that can have a profound effect on our health.

When purchasing natural hormone supplements or creams, keep the following in mind:

- More is not necessarily better. While some nutrients, such as vitamin C, can do more good therapeutically if you increase the dosages substantially, this is not the case with hormones. Always err on the side of caution, beginning with the lowest dosages and working your way up if needed.
- Read as much as you can about these hormones and why they may or may not benefit you. Remember, hormone supplementation is not for everyone. If you take time to evaluate your needs and educate yourself about the hormone(s) you are considering, you will feel much more comfortable with your final decision.
- As with any nutritional supplements, these hormones are not cure-alls or "youth in a bottle." It takes much more than swallowing a hormone to feel and look younger and healthier. If you want to feel and look younger longer, you will need a comprehensive approach that includes regular physical activity, a healthful diet, and a positive attitude.
- Treat these hormones with the respect they deserve. They may be able to provide incredible benefits, but proceed responsibly.

My personal experience

As a research journalist, I often like to experiment on myself. I am my own best guinea pig. I have had experience with three of the four over-the-counter hormones discussed in this chapter. Here is what I discovered (keep in mind that I am 35 years old):

- **Melatonin.** I have had inconsistent results using melatonin as a sleep aid. This is perhaps because of my age. I also believe my insomnia is not related to low melatonin production, but more possibly connected to the stress and deadlines I face each day. In addition, my Type-A personality probably doesn't help either. Regardless, I continue to try different melatonin products periodically.

- **DHEA.** At age 33, I had a complete hysterectomy due to ovarian cancer. Without testing my DHEA levels, I started taking the supplement to help with energy, mood, and menopausal relief. While I did notice an improvement in energy, I also started developing acne. As soon as I discontinued the DHEA, the acne disappeared. Since that time, I have had my DHEA levels tested. Not surprisingly, they are normal.

- **Progesterone.** I tend to agree with the experts who say progesterone is an overlooked and undervalued hormone supplement. Since I started using a progesterone cream, I have noticed a reduction in my menopausal symptoms. In addition, after reading the studies, I know I am supporting bone strength with this cream. New studies even suggest progesterone can help prevent breast cancer—and I am at very high risk for breast cancer due to a family history and my own cancer. I believe in this product and have become a walking progesterone testimonial.

I use my own experiences to help illustrate that we are all very separate individuals. What works for one person certainly may not work for another. You may have to experiment a bit. Once you find out what works best for you, you will be glad you were patient and took the time to investigate.

BUYER BE WISE

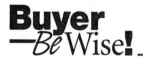

Chapter Five

Buying Other Natural Products

So many products, so little time! The vast number of choices available to us in the natural health industry can be mind boggling. So far, you've been given some general guidelines, learned about buying a multivitamin/mineral supplement, discovered the wonderful world of herbal medicine, and clarified the confusion about hormone supplements. In this chapter, we will tackle two more important categories—homeopathic medicines, and antioxidants. There is also information about glandular extracts.

Healing with homeopathy

While homeopathy is more than 200 years old, it is enjoying a resurgence of interest with today's baby boomers. At a time when healthcare costs are out of control, people are searching for more affordable alternatives. During their search, they find homeopathic medicines readily available over-the-counter. The new popularity is not surprising when you consider that homeopathy is very safe, inexpensive, and can be effective.

"Its appeal resides in that homeopathic medicines are gentle, noninvasive, and aid the body's own healing process rather than substituting for it," explains author and natural healthcare expert Michael Weiner, Ph.D.

"Homeopathy believes there is a vital force—an energy field—that, given the proper stimulation, can restore the physical, emotional, and mental equilibrium that has been disturbed by illness."

The homeopathic philosophy asserts that when the vital force is strong, the body can heal itself. Through a thorough analysis of the patient and the patient's symptoms, the homeopathic physician can choose the proper remedy. The remedy contains an extremely diluted form of ingredients. As much as 70 percent of the remedies are herbal in origin.

The homeopathic concept can be traced back as far as Hippocrates, who observed that when people took herbs in small doses, they cured the same symptoms they produced when given in large, toxic doses. This principle of homeopathy is called "like cures like," or the "law of similars."

Using a highly diluted remedy is one of the most controversial and hard-to-understand aspects of homeopathy. The idea is that the more the active compound of a certain substance (herb, vitamin, mineral, animal) is diluted, the better it works and the more powerful it becomes. The active ingredients in some homeopathic remedies are diluted so much that they are not recognized by current scientific equipment. This only encourages skepticism from the conventional medical community.

"Although such extreme dilution makes no sense in terms of Western medicine, it works," says Dr. Weiner.

One of the reasons it works, homeopathic practitioners say, is because it influences the body's energy systems. According to natural health writer and practitioner Kevon Arthurs, N.D., homeopathic medicines draw out the message of the plant or other substance that actually "speaks to the regulating energy systems of the body."

What about scientific validation? At least three of the world's leading research medical journals have published results supporting the effectiveness of homeopathy over a placebo (i.e., fake pill). One of the studies, evaluating people with hay fever, found that patients receiving a homeopathic remedy containing a mixture of grass pollen, suffered 50 percent fewer symptoms than the placebo group. Another study, with patients suffering from rheumatoid arthritis, found that 82 percent of the patients improved after taking a homeopathic remedy while only 21 percent of the placebo group improved. Still another study, featured in *The British Journal of Clinical Pharmacology*, showed that nearly twice as many flu patients, out of a total group of 487, recovered within 48 hours compared to those taking a placebo. The editors of the prominent journal *The Lancet* commended this study.

"Also, homeopathy has successfully treated infants and animals, where the placebo effect is highly unlikely," explains Dr. Weiner.

To better understand homeopathy, let's take a look at two key components of this unique form of medicine:

- **The principle of similars.** The idea that "like cures like" is the foundation of homeopathy. A thorough "picture" of symptoms is obtained and then matched with a remedy that actually would cause those symptoms in higher doses. Understandably, the potency or strength is matched with the seriousness of the illness.

- **Potency.** Homeopathic remedies are available in two basic categories of strength—x and c. The x remedies are made by diluting one part of the original material to nine parts of alcohol, water, or sugar. For example, a 12x remedy has been diluted 12 different times. The c remedies are considered to be more potent as they are diluted further. The c dilution dilutes one part of the material in 99 parts of the solution. This high dilution is believed to be not only stronger, but more "energized" or active.

For more clarification on this sometimes confusing topic, I contacted a leading authority on homeopathic medicines, Asa Hershoff, N.D., D.C.

Ask the Expert...Asa Hershoff, N.D., D.C.

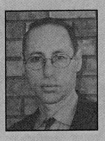 Dr. Asa Hershoff is a homeopath, naturopathic physician, and chiropractor. He has been in private practice for 24 years, currently at the California Homeopathic Clinic in Santa Monica. He was a founder of the Canadian College of Naturopathic Medicine and lectures and writes extensively.

KG—Why do you believe homeopathy provides people with a viable health option?

Dr. Hershoff—Each of the three main forms of natural medicine available to consumers— nutritional supplements, herbs, and homeopathy—has its own unique role to play in achieving and maintaining health. Homeopathy has an advantage of being virtually non-toxic and thus free of side effects or potential overdose. Homeopathic remedies have no known interaction or interference with other medicines, which cannot be said of vitamins or herbs. Their gentle action is particularly appropriate for children, the elderly, or those with a very sensitive metabolism. However, homeopathy is appropriate for everyone.

KG—It seems quite complex. How knowledgeable does a person have to be to use homeopathy?

Dr. Hershoff—Though using single homeopathic remedies requires a learning curve, the control and effectiveness it gives in overcoming simple health problems is well worth the investment of time and effort. On the other end of the spectrum, a trained and skilled professional homeopath can offer help for the full range of human ailments, including chronic, degenerative diseases. Additionally, homeopathy has a unique role to play in the treatment of mental and emotional conditions, as well as assisting deep psychological change and personal growth. With homeopathy, we want to reinforce and complement the body's attempt at healing—as expressed by symptoms—rather than suppress these reactions. In this lies the greatest distinction between homeopathy and mainstream medicine, which regards symptom-reactions as belonging to a mechanical disease process, rather than a dynamic curative response.

KG—We know there are two types of homeopathic products: single remedies and combination formulas. What is your opinion of each of these?

Dr. Hershoff—Single remedies are part of the *Homeopathic Pharmacoepia* of the United States, and they are prescribed to fit an exact set of symptoms. This allows a certain control and accuracy, but requires both accurate observation and a good working knowledge of the remedies. Combination remedies contain an assortment of the most frequently indicated remedies for a certain malady. The theory is that the body will use whichever remedy is most indicated and basically ignore the rest. Many classical homeopaths object to this approach. Nonetheless, combination remedies do generally work for acute and chronic conditions. Though they have not undergone homeopathic investigation or "provings", a number of these combination formulas have been medically researched. (*Note*: "Provings" are detailed records of symptoms.)

KG—Should consumers choose single remedies or combination formulas?

Dr. Hershoff—The conflict between classical homeopathy and the use of combination remedies can be resolved if it is realized that they each have their own value. It is not an "either/or" situation. Single remedies are essential for treating deep-seated illness, promoting a more comprehensive, holistic metabolic or psychological change, and altering deep patterns of disease susceptibility and tendency. Combination remedies are useful for the layperson for acute, local illness, or to promote the health of a particular organ, tissue, or process. In short, there is no substitute for an accurate "bull's eye" single remedy. However, a much faster, easier —even though it is somewhat less accurate—route is the use of the many combination remedies available.

KG—What should consumers watch out for when purchasing these combination formulas?

Dr. Hershoff—Homeopathic experience (and common sense) shows us that there are definite relationships among ingredients. Some complement each other, while others are antagonistic or counteract one another. A number of manufacturers, however, ignore this logic and combine remedies that have antidotal or even adverse effects when used together.

Here are some examples of combinations that should not be used together:
- Mercury and Silica
- *Rhus tox* and Apis
- *Nux vomica* tends to counteract many other remedies, especially those of plant origin
- Camphor also tends to counteract many other remedies

KG—How do consumers know if a formulation is bad?

Dr. Hershoff—Information on remedy relationships and compatibility can be found in homeopathic textbooks. To avoid choosing a "bad" product, combinations should not have too extensive a list of ingredients. Five or six is usually adequate to do the job and will help avoid unnecessary interactions among remedies. In addition, only one combination remedy or single remedy should be taken at a time. They may, however, be taken within a reasonable amount of time, usually a few hours apart.

KG—Can you help clarify some of the confusion over potencies of homeopathic remedies?

Dr. Hershoff—Potencies are a confusing issue for the health consumer. American and British homeopathic remedies are found in 6, 12, and 30 x or c. French manufacturers often use odd potencies such as 5, 9, and 15. While the question of potency is a complicated and controversial one, a simple rule of thumb can be applied. Lower strengths (lower numbers and x potencies) work for a shorter period of time, with less depth and on a more physical and material basis. Higher potencies (higher numbers and c potencies) work longer, deeper, and on a subtler level. In practice, 6 or 12 are good potencies for the beginner and will need to be repeated more frequently. The 30 strength is also very good and can be taken less often. High potencies like the 200, 1m, 10m, etc., should be left to experienced professionals.

KG—What should consumers look for when buying a homeopathic remedy?

Dr. Hershoff—Manufacturing itself is usually not an issue, as all homeopathic laboratories must be approved and monitored by the FDA. Still, use a brand that is known and trusted. There are far more combination manufacturers than single remedy manufacturers. Homeopathic remedies are sensitive creatures and must be packaged properly. I prefer glass containers versus plastic, even though some manufacturers claim their bottles are made of special, stable, non-degradable plastic. Containers must also be opaque, or if they are transparent, they should be completely covered by a label to prevent exposure to light. Tinted glass provides the best, most neutral type of container. Eye droppers should also be made of glass, not plastic (except for the bulb at the top, of course). Shelf life is indefinite for remedies in pellet form. Liquid remedies will eventually grow fungi, etc., after several months in spite of a certain amount of preserving alcohol. Keep homeopathic supplements out of intense heat or direct light. Keep them tightly closed and never open them around strong perfumes, incense, cooking odors, and so on.

KG—What are your thoughts on the different forms of homeopathic remedies?

Dr. Hershoff—If you are sensitive to alcohol or have a history of alcoholism, remedies should be taken in pill or tablet form. Most pellets are now made of sucrose, not lactose. People who are lactose intolerant are usually fine with pellets, but do check the label, especially with tablets. For the very sensitive, who do not even want this small amount of cane or milk sugar, the remedy can be opened and sniffed, and still produce reasonably good results.

KG—Is there a best form to take?

Dr. Hershoff—Unfortunately, research into the best form of delivery of homeopathic remedies has not been done to date. While remedies are generally taken by mouth, labels usually say that the remedy should be held under the tongue to help absorption. This is based on a misconception. Homeopathic remedies should be placed where there are rich nerve endings, which is on top of the tongue, not under it. The mouth should of course be free of foods or tastes when a remedy is taken. One of the oddest forms of homeopathic remedies comes in gelatin capsules and is swallowed like a regular vitamin. It seems unlikely these remedies would be effective in this manner.

KG—How important is the indication for use statement on the label of a homeopathic product?

Dr. Hershoff—One of the unfortunate (or bizarre, depending on how you look at it) facts about homeopathic products is that they are required by law to have a common indication on the label. Though the powers that be may have the public interest at heart, it is a misleading situation. In homeopathy, these remedies may be indicated for literally dozens of conditions or illnesses. Therefore, you may buy *Nux vomica* for your headache, but the label states "constipation" or "irritability." Similarly embarrassing is when I have prescribed *Pulsatilla* for a child's ear infection and the label says "vaginitis"! These indications should just be ignored. And again, you can ignore the expiration date, which is required by law. It has little relevance since remedies in pellet form can last over a century.

KG—Do you have any general warnings, cautions, or safety issues people should be aware of before buying homeopathic products?

Dr. Hershoff—Certain strengths and potencies should not be used by consumers, either in single remedies or combinations. These include potencies like the 200, 1m, 10m, or 50m. Because combination remedies are often used frequently or for a prolonged period of time, they should not contain deep-acting ingredients like *Lachesis, Naja, Staphylococcinum, Medorrhinum, Leusinum*, etc. In fact, over-the-counter homeopathic remedies should not, by law, contain these substances, but it does happen. The only homeopathic remedy listed in tests to be strictly avoided during pregnancy is called *Apis mellifica*. On the other hand, *Sepia*, from ink of the squid, has been known to cure every conceivable problem during pregnancy, from nausea to low back pain to toxemia. However, remedies should not be taken frivolously at this time, and the advice of a trained homeopath is always best.

KG—Any closing comments on this topic?

Dr. Hershoff—Once these few dynamics of homeopathy are understood, safe, effective and remarkably powerful homeopathic remedies will become an irreplaceable and invaluable resource for the home medicine chest. Once a mainstay of the early pioneers of this country, homeopathics are again finding their rightful place as one of the world's premier forms of natural, non-toxic medicines.

I have personally had great success with homeopathic medicines, specifically for insomnia and colds and flu. When we combine their impeccable safety record with consistent results, it's no wonder this unique form of medicine is experiencing a renewed popularity.

Another area of intense interest is supporting the body's immune system through the use of antioxidant nutrients. Let's take a closer look at this important topic.

Evaluating antioxidants

Our immune system can provide us with incredible protection against illness. It includes a complex array of organs, tissues, fluids, and cells sharing a common goal—to keep the human body healthy.

The immune system includes 54 billion white blood cells. They join forces with the countless macrophage, phagocyte, and other cells to ward off foreign invader cells. It is an intricate, internal army that works for you around the clock.

"The trillions of specialized warriors in our immune system are on 24-hour duty, vigilantly destroying and mopping up virus, bacteria, yeast, tumor cells, and toxins from both inside and outside the body and even dead cells," explains cancer expert Dr. Patrick Quillin in his comprehensive book, *Beating Cancer with Nutrition* (Nutrition Times Press, 1994). "When the immune system is not functioning at peak efficiency, we may get a cold or infection. And when the immune system is subdued for any extended period of time, cancer may result."

That's why keeping those immune system troops strong and alert should be a key objective of any health program. Unfortunately, at times this can be a challenging battle, considering the amount of free radicals waging war against us.

What are free radicals? No, they aren't political activists recently released from prison. They are the enemy of our immune system. Toxic free radicals are in the air we breathe, the water we drink, and the foods we eat. Free radicals enter our body and damage cells, potentially converting them into cancer cells or creating other debilitating diseases. When your immune system is overworked or weakened, it can't keep up with the elimination of free radicals.

Free-radical damage has been compared to rust on a car. As air hits the rusted metal, the problem spreads and ultimately causes a great deal of damage to the car. Sound pretty bleak? Fortunately, antioxidants act as the body's rust protectant. And that's why these special, immune-stimulating substances have been getting so much attention. Researchers believe antioxidant nutri-ents can help prevent illness, treat degenerative diseases, and may even slow the aging process.

Antioxidants are in foods and dietary supplements. They can actually shield our cells from free-radical dam-age. Antioxidants bolster an aggressive immune system response, allowing it to kill mutated cells and rid the body of toxic substances.

The "traditional," well-known antioxidants include vitamins C and E, beta-carotene, selenium, and zinc. However, science is confirming that there are many more antioxidant nutrients available to help keep our immune system strong.

The list of antioxidants is quite long; however, here are some of the more popular, newer antioxidants to enter the marketplace:

- Carotenoids (not only beta-carotene, but lyco-penes, lutein, etc.)
- Grape seed and pine bark extracts
- Green tea
- Lipoic acid
- CoQ10
- Garlic

Numerous other substances can also help stimulate the immune system. They include:

- Mushroom extracts
- Echinacea, goldenseal, and astragalus
- Glandular extracts such as spleen and thymus

Not surprisingly, there are many opinions on how we can keep our immune system healthy. However, remem-ber that it all begins with a balanced diet, regular exer-cise, and a positive attitude. Nutritional supplements should be used to complement healthy lifestyle choices.

Clearly, antioxidant nutrients are surfacing as key components to an immune-stimulating health program. Unfortunately, because there are so many choices, devel-oping a strong antioxidant foundation can be confusing and frustrating.

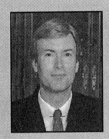
For clarification on this subject, I contacted Patrick Quillin, Ph.D., R.D., C.N.S. Dr. Quillin is a premier expert on immune system function.

KG—Will the new "high-tech" antioxidants take the place of the old "standbys" like vitamins C and E?

Dr. Quillin—No. Rather than replacing the "old standbys," these new antioxidants are providing us with a more complete picture of how our bodies work. We have several layers of antioxidant defenses, like the defensive team in football with a front line, middle linebackers, and defensive backs. We need all of those defenders intact in order to consider ourselves optimally protected against the continuous onslaught of free radicals. Given the fact that there are over 20,000 different bioflavonoids and 800 carotenoids in nature, plus millions of other substances in our complex food supply, I have no doubt that other valuable antioxidants are yet to be identified.

KG—With the excitement surrounding these antioxidant nutrients, what advice do you give people who want to start taking antioxidant products?

Dr. Quillin—Make sure you take a series of antioxidant nutrients in reasonable quantities and in as close to their natural state as possible. Nature provides us with an entire orchestra of antioxidants in a rich and varied food supply. These provide our bodies with several different layers of protection against oxidative damage. For instance, I take beta-carotene from algae, not as a synthetic chemical. I take multiple antioxidants simultaneously to ensure optimal protection, using such agents as bioflavonoids, vitamins C and E, selenium, and tocotrienols.

KG—Who needs antioxidant nutrients?

Dr. Quillin—All humans need a rich and diverse in-take of antioxidants throughout life. Yet, there are some factors that increase the need for antioxidants even further. These include vigorous exercise, smoking, alcohol intake, and chemotherapy and radiation (which work as pro-oxidants by increasing oxidation).

KG—What should consumers look for in an antioxidant supplement formulation?

Dr. Quillin—Balance, ratio, and source. While it is impossible to obtain all your antioxidants from natural food extracts, do so whenever you have the choice. For instance, vitamin C can be inexpensively manufactured from corn syrup and still provide us with essential antioxidant protection. Getting 1,000 mg of vitamin C daily from rose hips rather than synthetic vitamin C would require a 10-fold increase in spending and volume of pills. Meanwhile, other antioxidants, such as vitamin E and bioflavonoids, need to be taken in their natural state. Take reasonable amounts of antioxidants in the proper balance and from a high-quality source. You will be making a huge investment in a healthier future.

In his excellent book, *Beating Cancer with Nutrition*, Dr. Quillin provides us with this insight:

"While many very bright people have labored intensely, extensively, and expensively to develop some 'magic bullet' substance that would cure cancer, Nature has been patiently working on the same project for a couple of billion years...The more I study Nature and the human body, the more reverence I develop for the Great Engineer who designed us."

A word about glandular extracts

The same concept that governs the "law of similars" in homeopathy motivates glandular medicine—"like cures like." Glandular extracts are just that: extracts of mammalian glands. The glandular medicine philosophy believes that if a specific gland is ailing, you need to feed it that same glandular material. For example, an ill liver will benefit from raw liver extract.

Scientific evidence confirms the value of glandular therapy. Researchers have shown that these glands contain important enzymes, hormones, and other nutrients that can actually nourish the corresponding human gland. While the subject is controversial, these substances are present in many nutritional supplements.

The most common glandular extracts include liver, thymus, adrenal, thyroid, and spleen. However, nearly every gland in the human body has a corresponding glandular extract.

One of the most widely published glandular medicine testimonials comes from country singing sensation Naomi Judd. I had the pleasure of interviewing Naomi, an inspirational woman, about her battle with hepatitis C. This is the most serious, life-threatening form of hepatitis. In addition to many other important lifestyle and dietary changes, Naomi took a thymus extract supplement that has been tested against the hepatitis virus. She attributes her phenomenal recovery, in part, to this thymus extract.

Understandably, vegetarians avoid taking nutritional supplements that contain glandular extracts. The good news is that for every glandular extract on the market, there is typically a "vegan" alternative that is just as effective:

■ liver	↔	silymarin, dandelion, artichoke
■ adrenal	↔	ginseng, licorice, Mexican yam
■ thymus or spleen	↔	echinacea, goldenseal, antioxidant nutrients
■ thyroid	↔	iodine, kelp

So you see, while glandular therapy provides powerful medicine, vegetarians don't need to compromise their dietary standards to gain better health.

When reading the label of nutritional supplements with glandular extracts, recognize that many products do not give an exact milligram amount next to the glandular listing. These products will list the glandulars following the heading, "In a base of." This is not bad, but it does mean that the amount of glandular extract in the product may not be enough to provide a therapeutic or medicinal effect.

As with herbal extracts, many glandular extracts can be standardized for a specific component. For example, the thymus extract that Naomi Judd took was standardized for a specific peptide component of thymus tissue. This active compound was shown in scientific studies to provide the most positive influence on the human immune system.

Standardized glandular products should clearly identify the active ingredient and percentage of standardization. These glandular extracts are designed to treat a specific condition, and care should be taken when using them. A thyroid glandular extract taken at higher doses, for example, may have a negative impact on the health of susceptible individuals. Similar to hormone extracts, glandular supplements demand respect and caution. Do not exceed the recommended dosages and whenever possible, consult with a qualified healthcare professional.

Glandular extracts are still another viable alternative in the fascinating world of natural medicine.

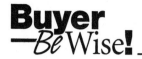
Putting it All Together

Is the term quality overused and undervalued? When it comes to nutritional supplements, I don't think so. Consumers, retailers, manufacturers, and researchers all recognize the value of quality when it comes to these health-promoting products.

Unfortunately, a few "shoddy" or even unscrupulous manufacturers, retailers, and researchers force us to be smart shoppers. This is true in any industry, not just the natural health field. Congratulations for taking the first step toward purchasing quality nutritional supplements. You are educating yourself and taking control.

Educational literature versus sales hype

The most important tool you can use to help you identify quality products—and the right products for your individual situation—is educational literature. Recognize that it can sometimes be difficult to distinguish true educational literature from product sales hype.

With the passage of looser legislation on nutritional supplements came the introduction of the "third-party literature" concept. According to the law, retailers, manufacturers, and distributors can disseminate information that makes claims for natural substances as long as the information is balanced, accurate, and not product-specific. The term "third party" indicates that the information was written or produced by a researcher, publisher, or reporter who has no financial-vested interest in the information presented. In other words, the source of the literature will not profit from the sale of a product with the ingredient(s) mentioned in the literature.

IMPAKT Communications, for example, is a third-party publisher because we do not gain any financial revenue from the sale of products with ingredients featured in our educational materials. Our only product is information. That's why it is so important for us to provide accurate, timely information that is trusted and respected. After all, if the information is not good, we no longer have an effective "product" to market.

Although retailers, distributors, and manufacturers sell products with ingredients mentioned in the educational literature, they can still share the literature if it is produced by a valid third party. Retailers, distributors, and manufacturers are not allowed by law to produce educational literature that makes claims for many of the products or ingredients they sell. They must obtain their educational literature from third-party sources.

Let's take a look at ways you can distinguish true educational literature from sales/promotional materials. The types of literature you will be evaluating include magazines, books, booklets, and article reprints. Credible literature means it should be:

■ Written by healthcare professionals or qualified research journalists.
■ Published by a publisher with no product ties.
■ Balanced, with information about toxicity and contraindications.
■ Comprehensive, including information about dosages and applications.
■ Fact, not fiction or merely opinion.

Here are some red flags that may indicate the information is not truly third-party educational literature:

■ A byline by someone with a financial interest in the product(s) or ingredient(s) mentioned in the article.

- No sources (i.e., books, magazines, medical journals, other experts, or references) given in the literature.
- The publisher or source of publication is not identified.
- An obvious sales slant or the mention of specific product names.
- The words "miracle" or "cure" should be used sparingly, if at all. (Respected author Jean Carper obviously disagrees with this caution as she named her latest book, *Miracle Cures*. Oh, well, I guess it's a matter of journalistic opinion.)

Analyze the educational literature you receive just as carefully as you investigate the nutritional supplements you are considering. Remember, the two go hand-in-hand.

Our editor, Frances FitzGerald, explained it best in a letter that was printed in *USA Today* (12/3/97), following an article they published on herbal medicine: "Consumers need to find unbiased, third-party sources who are independent of any manufacturer. Only then can they be sure of getting objective facts rather than a sales pitch...by finding accurate, balanced information on these compounds, consumers can reap their full benefits."

"There is no substitute for knowledge..." explains Jean Carper in her best-selling book, *Miracle Cures*. "Obviously, the more you know about natural remedies, in particular the ones you are interested in using, the better. And the more serious the disease you are attempting to treat, the more care you must exercise and the more you must know."

Information is power. It will help you protect your most critical asset: your health.

You deserve the very best

In a well-known hair color commercial, a beautiful blond model brushes her hair back, confidently proclaiming "because I'm worth it!" When it comes to your health, you deserve the best. Remember, you're worth it!

I have personally experienced the devastation of disease. Within an eight-month period, my sister was diagnosed with breast cancer, my mom died just three weeks after discovering she had advanced pancreatic cancer, and I was operated on for ovarian cancer. During that time, I learned a valuable lesson: We need to do everything we can to protect our health and the health of those we love. We have a plethora of products available to help us accomplish this goal. By doing the proper research before the purchase, we have a much better chance of buying quality products that enhance our health.

There is no question that it takes a certain amount of "wisdom" to buy the right products. Now that you have gained the wisdom from some of the most respected experts in the natural health industry, you should feel more confident and comfortable in making your supplement purchases. But remember, it's a never-ending process of continual education and information. Enjoy the journey!

Final quotes and comments...

"Fortunately, the attitude toward natural treatments is rapidly changing in the United States. More scientific information on natural remedies is coming into the country; prestigious scientists and doctors here are increasingly testing and using such natural remedies and comparing their effectiveness and safety with pharmaceutical drugs. And Americans are embracing the natural medications and so-called 'alternative' or 'complementary' treatments with enthusiasm."
—Jean Carper, *Miracle Cures* (Harper Collins, 1997)

"Research evaluating the cost and clinical effectiveness of utilizing natural medicine practices, replacing drugs with natural medicines, and combining natural medicine with conventional medicine has concluded that these practices promote health and decrease costs."
—Joseph Pizzorno, *Total Wellness* (Prima, 1996)

"Health is wholeness and balance, an inner resilience that allows you to meet the demands of living without being overwhelmed. If you have that kind of resilience, you can experience the inevitable interactions with germs and not get infections, you can be in contact with allergens and not suffer allergies, and you can sustain exposure to carcinogens and not get cancer. Optimal health should also bring with it a sense of strength and joy, so that you experience it as more than just the absence of disease."
—Andrew Weil, M.D., *8 Weeks to Optimum Health* (Knopf, 1997)

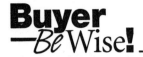

Recommended reading

Books by the experts

- *Beating Cancer with Nutrition*
  by Patrick Quillin, Ph.D., R.D., C.N.S.
  254 pages $14.95 (U.S.) $20.20 (Canada)

- *DHEA: A Practical Guide*
  by Ray Sahelian, M.D.
  158 pages $9.95 (U.S.) $13.95 (Canada)

- *The Green Pharmacy*
  by James Duke, Ph.D.
  507 pages $29.95 (U.S.) $41.95 (Canada)

- *Homeopathy for Musculoskeletal Healing*
  by Asa Hershoff, N.D., D.C.
  314 pages $20.00 (U.S.) $28.00 (Canada)

- *Hormone Replacement: An Individualized Approach*
  by Marla Ahlgrimm, R.Ph., and John Kells
  38 pages $3.95 (U.S.) $5.35 (Canada)

- *Melatonin: Nature's Sleeping Pill*
  by Ray Sahelian, M.D.
  144 pages $9.95 (U.S.) $13.95 (Canada)

- *Pregnenolone*
  by Ray Sahelian, M.D.
  157 pages $9.95 (U.S.) $13.95 (Canada)

- *Preventing and Reversing Osteoporosis*
  by Alan Gaby, M.D.
  304 pages $14.95 (U.S.) $26.95 (Canada)

- *Saw Palmetto: Nature's Prostate Healer*
  by Ray Sahelian, M.D.
  150 pages $5.99 (U.S.) $7.50 (Canada)

- *The Vitamin Revolution in Health Care*
  by Michael Janson, M.D.
  236 pages $12.95 (U.S.) $17.95 (Canada)

For a free catalog of books published and distributed by IMPAKT Communications, send your request with your name and address to:

IMPAKT Communications
P.O. Box 12496
Green Bay, WI 54307-2496

Quantity discounts for *Buyer Be Wise!* are available by calling 1-800-477-2995.

Your comments are appreciated:
e-mail = impakt@dct.com
or visit our web site at www.impakt.com

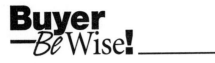

Glossary/Index

"The art of healing comes from nature and not from the physician. Therefore, the physician must start from nature with an open mind."
—Paracelsus, 16th century Swiss physician

IMPAKT Health Series Booklets

*Ray Sahelian, M.D., answers your questions
on some of the hottest topics.*

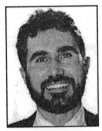

Ray Sahelian, M.D.,
is also the author of
best-selling books on
*Melatonin, DHEA,
Creatine, Glucosamine*
and *Pregnenolone,* and
is editor of *Longevity
Research Update.*

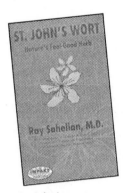

St. John's wort
Paperback • 32 pp
$4.00

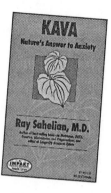

Kava
Paperback • 32 pp
$4.00

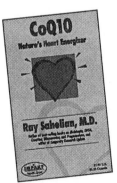

CoQ10
Paperback • 32 pp
$4.00

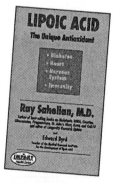

Lipoic Acid
Paperback • 30 pp
$4.00

Available by calling 1-800-477-2995.

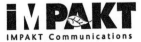

IMPAKT Communications